TAI CHI SECRETS OF THE WU STYLE

Tai Chi Secrets of the Wu Style

Chinese Classics • Translations • Commentary

by Dr. Yang, Jwing-Ming

YMAA Publication Center
Wolfeboro, NH USA

YMAA Publication Center
Main Office:
  PO Box 480
  Wolfeboro, NH, 03894 USA
  800-669-8892 • info@ymaa.com • www.ymaa.com

20200226

Edited by James O'Leary

Cover design by Katya Popova

ISBN 13: 978-1-886969-17-9
ISBN 10: 1-886969-17-5

Publisher's Cataloging in Publication
(Prepared by Quality Books Inc.)

Yang, Jwing-Ming, 1946-
    Tai chi secrets of the Wu style : Chinese classics,
translations, commentary / by Yang, Jwing-Ming. — 1st
ed.
        p. cm.
        Includes index.
        Chiefly in English; some text in Chinese.
        LCCN: 2002101587
        ISBN: 1-886969-17-5

        1. Tai chi.   I. Title.

GV504.Y36 2002   613.7'148
                                  QBI02-200165

Printed in USA.

Contents

Foreword

The content of Chinese Wushu (武術)(martial arts) is vast and highly diverse. Various schools and styles of Wushu are often categorized into the internal and external varieties. Taijiquan is one of the major divisions of the internal school. Within Taijiquan there are dozens of sub-categories based on the teachings of one Master or a family with gen- 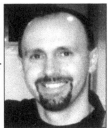 erations of experts. The origins of some forms are well documented and reference material is readily available. The Chen (陳) and Yang (楊) styles which precede the other forms historically have dozens of videotapes, vcd publications, and printed materials available in several languages. Of the five primary family styles of Taijiquan, the Wu style (吳氏) is not as widely practiced in the West as the other forms. Noted for compact structure, gentle and fluid movements, and beautiful balancing techniques, Wu style Taijiquan can provide a solid foundation in many areas: fitness, healing, recreation, personal devel-opment and effective self-defense training. The practitioner must have some clear understanding of the basic tenets of the art in order to develop real skills, hence the necessity for the transmission of the essential information by the true Masters of the art. Unfortunately, published material on this style is especially difficult to find.

Tai Chi Secrets of Wu Style by Dr. Yang, Jwing-Ming promises to be a major source of information on this beautiful and useful martial art. In this work, Dr. Yang has included the English transla-tion as well as the original Chinese text, enabling us to examine the material from both language perspectives. Although I have studied martial arts more than thirty years, my limited experience with Wu style leads me to welcome the chance to explore the essence of Wu, Jian-Quan's (吳鑑泉) teaching. For many years Dr. Yang's work has informed and inspired martial artists around the world. His transla-tions and insightful commentary afford us the opportunity to delve deeply into the theories and philosophies of prior generations. The Chinese martial arts practitioners of the West owe a great debt of gratitude to Dr. Yang for this and his many other contributions to the development and promotion of our art. There is a famous saying among Chinese Wushu people which begins: "Shifu Ling Jin men." (師父領進門) (The teacher leads into the door.) Dr. Yang, Jwing-Ming has opened many doors for us. This portal to the essence of the Wu style Taijiquan traditions provides access to hitherto unavailable information, yet again expanding the boundaries of the Chinese martial world.

Nick Gracenin
July 7, 2001

About the Author

Dr. Yang, Jwing-Ming, Ph.D. 楊俊敏博士

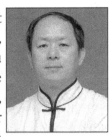

Dr. Yang, Jwing-Ming was born on August 11th, 1946, in Xinzhu Xian (新竹縣), Taiwan (台灣), Republic of China (中華民國). He started his Wushu (武術)(Gongfu or Kung Fu, 功夫) training at the age of fifteen under the Shaolin White Crane (Bai He, 少林白鶴) Master Cheng, Gin-Gsao (曾金灶). Master Cheng originally learned Taizuquan (太祖拳) from his grandfather when he was a child. When Master Cheng was fifteen years old, he started learning White Crane from Master Jin, Shao-Feng (金紹峰), and followed him for twenty-three years until Master Jin's death.

In thirteen years of study (1961-1974 A.D.) under Master Cheng, Dr. Yang became an expert in the White Crane Style of Chinese martial arts, which includes both the use of barehands and of various weapons such as saber, staff, spear, trident, two short rods, and many other weapons. With the same master he also studied White Crane Qigong (氣功), Qin Na (or Chin Na, 擒拿), Tui Na (推拿) and Dian Xue massages (點穴按摩), and herbal treatment.

At the age of sixteen, Dr. Yang began the study of Yang Style Taijiquan (楊氏太極拳) under Master Kao Tao (高濤). After learning from Master Kao, Dr. Yang continued his study and research of Taijiquan with several masters and senior practitioners such as Master Li, Mao-Ching (李茂清) and Mr. Wilson Chen (陳威伸) in Taipei (台北). Master Li learned his Taijiquan from the well-known Master Han, Ching-Tang (韓慶堂), and Mr. Chen learned his Taijiquan from Master Zhang, Xiang-San (張祥三). Dr. Yang has mastered the Taiji barehand sequence, pushing hands, the two-man fighting sequence, Taiji sword, Taiji saber, and Taiji Qigong.

When Dr. Yang was eighteen years old he entered Tamkang College (淡江學院) in Taipei Xian to study Physics. In college he began the study of traditional Shaolin Long Fist (Changquan or Chang Chuan, 少林長拳) with Master Li, Mao-Ching at the Tamkang

College Guoshu Club (淡江國術社)(1964-1968 A.D.), and eventually became an assistant instructor under Master Li. In 1971 he completed his M.S. degree in Physics at the National Taiwan University (台灣大學), and then served in the Chinese Air Force from 1971 to 1972. In the service, Dr. Yang taught Physics at the Junior Academy of the Chinese Air Force (空軍幼校) while also teaching Wushu. After being honorably discharged in 1972, he returned to Tamkang College to teach Physics and resumed study under Master Li, Mao-Ching. From Master Li, Dr. Yang learned Northern Style Wushu, which includes both barehand (especially kicking) techniques and numerous weapons.

In 1974, Dr. Yang came to the United States to study Mechanical Engineering at Purdue University. At the request of a few students, Dr. Yang began to teach Gongfu (Kung Fu), which resulted in the foundation of the Purdue University Chinese Kung Fu Research Club in the spring of 1975. While at Purdue, Dr. Yang also taught college-credited courses in Taijiquan. In May of 1978 he was awarded a Ph.D. in Mechanical Engineering by Purdue.

In 1980, Dr. Yang moved to Houston to work for Texas Instruments. While in Houston he founded Yang's Shaolin Kung Fu Academy, which was eventually taken over by his disciple Mr. Jeffery Bolt after moving to Boston in 1982. Dr. Yang founded Yang's Martial Arts Academy (YMAA) in Boston on October 1, 1982.

In January of 1984 he gave up his engineering career to devote more time to research, writing, and teaching. In March of 1986 he purchased property in the Jamaica Plain area of Boston to be used as the headquarters of the new organization, Yang's Martial Arts Association. The organization has continued to expand, and, as of July 1st 1989, YMAA has become just one division of Yang's Oriental Arts Association, Inc. (YOAA, Inc.).

In summary, Dr. Yang has been involved in Chinese Wushu since 1961. During this time, he has spent thirteen years learning Shaolin White Crane (Bai He), Shaolin Long Fist (Changquan), and Taijiquan. Dr. Yang has more than thirty-three years of instructional experience: seven years in Taiwan, five years at Purdue University, two years in Houston, Texas, and nineteen years in Boston, Massachusetts.

In addition, Dr. Yang has also been invited to offer seminars around the world to share his knowledge of Chinese martial arts and Qigong. The countries he has visited include Argentina, Austria, Barbados, Belgium, Bermuda, Botswana, Canada, Chile, England, France, Germany, Holland, Hungary, Ireland, Italy, Latvia, Mexico, Poland, Portugal, Saudi Arabia, Spain, South Africa, Switzerland, and Venezuela.

Since 1986, YMAA has become an international organization, which currently includes 52 schools located in Argentina, Belgium, Canada, Chile, England, France, Holland, Hungary, Iran, Ireland, Italy, Poland, Portugal, South Africa, Spain, Venezuela and the United States. Many of Dr. Yang's books and videotapes have been translated into languages such as French, Italian, Spanish, Polish, Czech, Bulgarian, Russian, Hungarian, and Persian.

Dr. Yang has published twenty-nine other volumes on the martial arts and *Qigong*:

1. *Shaolin Chin Na;* Unique Publications, Inc., 1980.
2. *Shaolin Long Fist Kung Fu;* Unique Publications, Inc., 1981.
3. *Yang Style Tai Chi Chuan;* Unique Publications, Inc., 1981.
4. *Introduction to Ancient Chinese Weapons;* Unique Publications, Inc., 1985.
5. *Qigong for Health and Martial Arts;* YMAA Publication Center, 1985.
6. *Northern Shaolin Sword;* YMAA Publication Center, 1985.
7. *Tai Chi Theory and Martial Power;* YMAA Publication Center, 1986.
8. *Tai Chi Chuan Martial Applications;* YMAA Publication Center, 1986.
9. *Analysis of Shaolin Chin Na;* YMAA Publication Center, 1987.
10. *Eight Simple Qigong Exercises for Health;* YMAA Publication Center, 1988.
11. *The Root of Chinese Qigong—The Secrets of Qigong Training;* YMAA Publication Center, 1989.

12. *Muscle/Tendon Changing and Marrow/Brain Washing Chi Kung—The Secret of Youth*; YMAA Publication Center, 1989.

13. *Hsing Yi Chuan—Theory and Applications*; YMAA Publication Center, 1990.

14. *The Essence of Taiji Qigong—Health and Martial Arts*; YMAA Publication Center, 1990.

15. *Qigong for Arthritis*; YMAA Publication Center, 1991.

16. *Chinese Qigong Massage—General Massage*; YMAA Publication Center, 1992.

17. *How to Defend Yourself*; YMAA Publication Center, 1992.

18. *Baguazhang—Emei Baguazhang*; YMAA Publication Center, 1994.

19. *Comprehensive Applications of Shaolin Chin Na—The Practical Defense of Chinese Seizing Arts*; YMAA Publication Center, 1995.

20. *Taiji Chin Na—The Seizing Art of Taijiquan*; YMAA Publication Center, 1995.

21. *The Essence of Shaolin White Crane*; YMAA Publication Center, 1996.

22. *Back Pain—Chinese Qigong for Healing and Prevention*; YMAA Publication Center, 1997.

23. *Ancient Chinese Weapons*; YMAA Publication Center, 1999.

24. *Taijiquan—Classical Yang Style*; YMAA Publication Center, 1999.

25. *Tai Chi Secrets of Ancient Masters*; YMAA Publication Center, 1999.

26. *Taiji Sword—Classical Yang Style*; YMAA Publication Center, 1999.

27. *Tai Chi Secrets of Wŭ & Li Styles*; YMAA Publication Center, 2001.

28. *Tai Chi Secrets of Yang Style*; YMAA Publication Center, 2001.

29. *Tai Chi Secrets of Wu Style*; YMAA Publication Center, 2002.

Dr. Yang has also published the following videotapes:

1. *Yang Style Tai Chi Chuan and Its Applications*; YMAA Publication Center, 1984.
2. *Shaolin Long Fist Kung Fu—Lien Bu Chuan and Its Applications*; YMAA Publication Center, 1985.
3. *Shaolin Long Fist Kung Fu—Gung Li Chuan and Its Applications*; YMAA Publication Center, 1986.
4. *Shaolin Chin Na*; YMAA Publication Center, 1987.
5. *Wai Dan Chi Kung, Vol. 1—The Eight Pieces of Brocade*; YMAA Publication Center, 1987.
6. *The Essence of Tai Chi Chi Kung*; YMAA Publication Center, 1990.
7. *Qigong for Arthritis*; YMAA Publication Center, 1991.
8. *Qigong Massage—Self Massage*; YMAA Publication Center, 1992.
9. *Qigong Massage—With a Partner*; YMAA Publication Center, 1992.
10. *Defend Yourself 1—Unarmed Attack*; YMAA Publication Center, 1992.
11. *Defend Yourself 2—Knife Attack*; YMAA Publication Center, 1992.
12. *Comprehensive Applications of Shaolin Chin Na 1*; YMAA Publication Center, 1995.
13. *Comprehensive Applications of Shaolin Chin Na 2*; YMAA Publication Center, 1995.
14. *Shaolin Long Fist Kung Fu—Yi Lu Mai Fu & Er Lu Mai Fu*; YMAA Publication Center, 1995.
15. *Shaolin Long Fist Kung Fu—Shi Zi Tang*; YMAA Publication Center, 1995.
16. *Taiji Chin Na*; YMAA Publication Center, 1995.
17. *Emei Baguazhang—1; Basic Training, Qigong, Eight Palms, and Applications*; YMAA Publication Center, 1995.
18. *Emei Baguazhang—2; Swimming Body Baguazhang and Its Applications*; YMAA Publication Center, 1995.

19. *Emei Baguazhang—3; Bagua Deer Hook Sword and Its Applications*; YMAA Publication Center, 1995.
20. *Xingyiquan—12 Animal Patterns and Their Applications*; YMAA Publication Center, 1995.
21. *24 and 48 Simplified Taijiquan*; YMAA Publication Center, 1995.
22. *White Crane Hard Qigong*; YMAA Publication Center, 1997.
23. *White Crane Soft Qigong*; YMAA Publication Center, 1997.
24. *Xiao Hu Yan—Intermediate Level Long Fist Sequence*; YMAA Publication Center, 1997.
25. *Back Pain—Chinese Qigong for Healing and Prevention*; YMAA Publication Center, 1997.
26. *Scientific Foundation of Chinese Qigong*; YMAA Publication Center, 1997.
27. *Taijiquan—Classical Yang Style*; YMAA Publication Center, 1999.
28. *Taiji Sword—Classical Yang Style*; YMAA Publication Center, 1999.
29. *Chin Na in Depth—1*; YMAA Publication Center, 2000.
30. *Chin Na in Depth—2*; YMAA Publication Center, 2000.
31. *San Cai Jian & Its Applications*; YMAA Publication Center, 2000.
32. *Kun Wu Jian & Its Applications*; YMAA Publication Center, 2000.
31. *Qi Men Jian & Its Applications*; YMAA Publication Center, 2000.
34. *Chin Na in Depth—3*; YMAA Publication Center, 2001.
35. *Chin Na in Depth—4*; YMAA Publication Center, 2001.
36. *Chin Na in Depth—5*; YMAA Publication Center, 2001.

37. *Chin Na in Depth—6*; YMAA Publication Center, 2001.
38. *Shaolin Long Fist Kung Fu—Twelve Tan Tui & Their Applications*; YMAA Publication Center, 2001.

Introduction

In the last seven centuries, many songs and poems have been composed about Taijiquan. These have played a major role in preserving the knowledge and wisdom of the masters, although in many cases the identity of the authors and the dates of origin have been lost. Since most Chinese of previous centuries were illiterate, the key points of the art were put into poems and songs, which are easier to remember than prose, and passed down orally from teacher to student. They were regarded as secret and have only been revealed to the general public in this century.

It is very difficult to translate these ancient Chinese writings. Because of the cultural differences, many expressions would not make sense to the Westerner if translated literally. Often, knowledge of the historical context is necessary. Furthermore, since in Chinese different sounds can have several possible meanings, through the decades when anyone tried to understand a poem or write it down, he would have to choose from among these meanings. For this reason, many of the poems have several variations. The same problem occurs when the poems are read. Many Chinese characters have several possible meanings, so reading involves interpretation of the text even for the Chinese. Also, the meaning of many words has changed over the course of time. When you add to this the grammatical differences (generally no tenses, articles, singular or plural, or differentiation between parts of speech) you find that it is almost impossible to translate ancient Chinese literally into English. In addition to all this, the translator must have much the same experience and understanding, as well as similar intuitive feelings as the original author, in order to convey the same meaning.

With these difficulties in mind, the author has attempted to convey as much of the original meaning of the Chinese as possible, based on his own Taiji experience and understanding. Although it is impossible to totally translate the original meaning, the author feels he has managed to express the majority of the important points. The translation has been made as close to the original Chinese as possible, including such things as double negatives and, sometimes, idiosyncratic sentence structure. Words that are understood but not actually written in the Chinese text have been included in parentheses. Also, some Chinese words are followed by the English in parentheses, e.g. Shen (Spirit). To further assist the reader, the author has included commentary with each poem and song.

In order to help the Taijiquan practitioner understand the essence of Taijiquan and its root, the author intends to translate the existing and available ancient Taijiquan documents from various sources. This includes the secrets of many well known ancient masters such as Zhang, San-Feng (張三豐), and Wang, Zong-Yue (王宗岳), as well as other, unknown authors. This includes the secrets of different Taijiquan styles well-known today, such as Yang (楊), Wu (吳), and Chen (陳). This continues the work the author began in the book, *Tai Chi Secrets of the Ancient Masters*, which will be further continued in forthcoming books on the secrets of Yang's family and Chen's family.

Included in this book are nineteen of the most typically available documents regarding Wu's family. Most of this information was obtained from the book, *The Lecture of Taijiquan*, (太極拳講義), by Wu, Gong-Zao (吳公藻) published in 1935, Shanghai, China. In addition, there is a foreword written for this book by another Taijiquan master, Xiang, Kai-Ran (向愷然), which is included in Appendix A. This foreword is included simply because it covers many common questions and answers which may untie many doubts for Taijiquan practitioners.

About Wu Style Taijiquan

Wu Style Taijiquan (吳氏太極拳) was created by Wu, Quan-You (吳全佑)(1834-1902) who learned Taijiquan from Yang, Ban-Hou (楊班候)(1837-1892), the second son of Yang Style creator, Yang, Lu-Shan (楊露禪)(1799-1872). Wu, Quan-You passed his art down to his son, Wu, Jian-Quan (吳鑑泉)(1870-1942). After learning from his father, Wu, Jian-Quan continued to modify the style until it became today's Wu Style Taijiquan.

Wu, Jian-Quan had two sons, Wu, Gong-Yi (吳公儀) and Wu, Gong-Zao (吳公藻), and two daughters, Wu, Ying-Hua (吳英華) and Wu, Jun-Hua (吳俊華). All of his children inherited the traditional teaching and training of the Wu style. This also included Wu, Jian-Quan's son-in-law, Ma, Yue-Liang (馬岳梁). Ma, Yue-Liang was well-known and a great Wu style promoter at the early time of Wu style development.

Today, Wu Style Taijiquan has become popular both in Asia and the Western world, and is now recognized as one of the four major styles of Taijiquan. These four styles are: Yang (楊), Chen (陳), Wu (吳), and Sun (孫).

Thanks to Erik Elsemans for proofing the manuscript and contributing many valuable suggestions and discussions. Thanks to Katya Popova for the cover design. Also, thanks to the editor, James O'Leary.

The Total Thesis of Taijiquan

太極拳總論

The Dao of the fist techniques (i.e., martial arts) is no more than strengthening the tendons and bones (i.e., physical body), and regulate and harmonize the Qi and the blood. However, Taijiquan follows the theory of the Taiji's movements and calmness as the methods (i.e., rules or theory), uses the marvelous variations of the insubstantial and substantial as the applications. Its postures are centered, upright, peaceful, and comfortable. Its movements are light, agile, round, and alive. Therefore, once moves, there is nothing without movement, once calm, there is nothing without calmness. Its theory of movements and calmness is consistent with the sitting Gong (i.e., sitting meditation) of the Dao's family (i.e., Daoism). In fact, it is the moving Gong (i.e., Qigong) of the Daoist family. (Therefore), from the viewpoint of the fist theory (i.e., martial theory), it can be called "internal family." It is because it contains the same body (i.e., same root and theoretical foundation) of the Dao.

拳術一道，不外強健筋骨，調和氣血。而太極拳，乃循太極動靜之理以為法，採虛實變化之妙而為用。其姿勢也中正安舒，其動作也輕靈圓活。故一動無有不動，一靜無有不靜。其動靜之理，與道家之坐功，互相吻合，實道家之行功。在拳理言之故稱內家，因與道本為一體。

Fist Techniques (Quan Shu, 拳術) is the general term for martial arts. The main purpose of training martial arts, other than self-defense, is to strengthen the physical body and to improve the circulation of the Qi and blood. Taijiquan was created in the Daoist monastery located in Wudang mountain (武當山) of Hubei (湖北) Province. It

1

was developed based on the Taiji Yin-Yang theory recorded in *Yi Jing* (*Book of Change*, 易經) which was created more than three thousand years ago (around 1122 B.C.). Therefore Taijiquan theory adopts the Yin-Yang concepts of movement (Yang) and calmness (Yin) as the main training methods. In addition, it uses the theory of insubstantial (Yin) and substantial (Yang) strategic movements as the foundation of the martial maneuvers and applications.

In order to be relaxed and allow the Qi to circulate smoothly, the torso is upright, natural, and comfortable. The movements are round, relaxed, agile, smooth, and alive. Because of these conditions, the entire body acts as a single unit. Once there is movement, the entire body moves, and once there is stillness (or the movement stops), the entire body is still. This theory of movement and calmness, and also the internal and external cultivations that implement it, are consistent with Daoist theory. This is because, as in sitting meditation, the cultivations emphasize the same principles and practices of regulating the body (Tiao Shen, 調身), breathing (Tiao Xi, 調息), mind (Tiao Xin, 調心), Qi (Tiao Qi, 調氣), and spirit (Tiao Shen, 調神). Thus, Taijiquan can be accurately described as moving meditation, as well as an internal martial style (i.e., Nei Jia, 內家). In fact, Taijiquan belongs to the Dao and the Dao contains Taijiquan. They are closely related to each other.

What are the movements and calmness? (It) is executing the original (thinking) of the Yi (i.e., wisdom mind). What are the insubstantial and substantial? It is the foundation of applying the Jins (i.e., martial power). Hidden internally is Jin, it is the main body (i.e., main content). Those manifested externally are postures and are the applications (of the internal). Use the calmness to govern the movements, and search for the movements in the calmness. Use the softness to subdue the hardness, and use the hardness to support the softness. To accept adversity philosophically and follow nature instinctively. This can be done because the feeling makes it so. Feel in the body and awareness (i.e., understand) in the heart (i.e., mind). (Whenever) the body feels, the heart (is immediately) aware. Listen (i.e., Gauge) its insubstantial and substantial and request (i.e., testing) its movement and stillness. (Once I) have gained the opponent's center, then I investigate myself and gauge the opponent. Use the opportunity and situation, exchange (my) insubstantial and substantial to attack and defeat (my opponent).

動靜者，行意之本源。虛實者，運勁之基礎。蘊之
於內者曰勁，以為體。形之於外者曰勢，以為用。
以靜制動，動中求靜。以柔克剛，剛以濟柔。逆來
順受，任其自然。蓋由於感覺使然。感之於身，覺
之於心。身有所感，心有所覺。聽其虛實，問其動
靜。得其重心，然後審己量敵，運用機勢，變換虛
實，攻而取之。

Your movement and calmness are initiated from your Yi (意)(i.e., wisdom mind). The mind then leads the Qi to the physical body for action. It is also your mind that makes the insubstantial and substantial strategic actions. Therefore, the mind's insubstantial and substantial is the foundation of the Jin's manifestation. The mind and the Qi generated internally are called Internal Jin (Nei Jin, 內勁). When Nei Jin is manifested into external postures, it is called External Jin (Wai Jin, 外勁). Therefore, those Jins that develop internally are the main body of the Jin's formation. Only when this internal Jin is manifested externally, can it be said that the Jin is completed.

Use defensive actions for offense. In order to execute this strategy effectively, mental calmness is the first crucial key. Even within the movements, internal calmness remains most important. When you are calm, the mind can be clear and your actions can be precise and firm. Softness and hardness are mutually exchangeable and support each other. In order to be connected, you must learn to be soft and follow the opponent's force naturally. Only then can you lead and neutralize the incoming force into emptiness. Success in this depends on how sensitively you can feel (i.e., Listening Jin) the opponent, and see through his intention.

When the body is touched, the mind immediately responds, gauging the opponent's insubstantial and substantial and investigating his center. After knowing your opponent and evaluating your capability, exploit any advantageous timing and condition, and skillfully exchange your insubstantial and substantial. When all of this happens, you have grasped the key to victory.

The classic says: "Although in techniques, there are many side doors (i.e., other martial art styles), after all, it is nothing more than the strong beating the weak." Also says: "Investigate (consider) the saying of four ounces repel one thousand pounds. It is apparent that this cannot be accomplished by strength." That the strong beating the weak is due to the pre-birth natural capability which is born with it. It (the capability) is not obtained from learning. What is called "using the four ounces to repel one thousand pounds" is actually matching the theory of using the balance (i.e., leverage). It does not matter the lightness or the heaviness of the body, the large or small of the force, can shift the opponent's weighting center, and (finally) move his entire body. Therefore, the reason that the movements of Taijiquan are different from other (martial) techniques, is because they do not defeat the opponent with force. Furthermore, (it) can not only strengthen the tendons, keep the bone healthy, and harmonize the Qi and blood, but can also be used to cultivate (i.e., harmonize) the body and (mental) mind, keep away from sickness and extend the life. (It) is a marvelous Dao of post-heaven body cultivation.

經云：〝斯技旁門甚多，概不外有力打無力。〞又
曰：〝查四兩撥千斤之句，顯非力勝。〞夫有力打
無力，斯乃先天自然之能，生而知之。非學而後能
之。所謂四兩撥千斤者，實則合乎權衡之理。無論
體之輕重，力之大小，能在動之間，移其重心，使
之全身牽動。故太極拳之動作，所以異於他技者，
非務以力勝人也。推而進之，不惟強筋健骨，調和
氣血，而自能修養身心，卻病延年，為後天養身之
妙道焉。

Taijiquan emphasizes softness to counter hardness, and also uses
the idea of four ounces to repel one thousand pounds to express
the concept of early, gradual and precise interception rather than
so-called "dumb" blocking (hard, stiff blocks). In order to reach this
level of skill, you must learn how to exploit the dynamics of balance. If you can protect your balance and center, and at the same
time move the opponent's balance off and shift his center, you will
put your opponent into a disadvantageous situation for your further
action. Only if you can use your balanced force to lead the opponent
into imbalance can you neutralize the incoming thousand pounds of
force with just a little force.

Moreover, since Taijiquan emphasizes softness, the entire body
and especially the joints must be relaxed, so that the Qi can be led
by the mind efficiently and smoothly. These practices can not only
improve your mental concentration, but also help to harmonize the
Qi and blood to improve physical health.

The Important Meaning of Taijiquan Thirteen Postures

太
極
拳
十
三
勢
大
義

The thirteen postures, (are derived) according to the theory of five elements and eight trigrams. They are the thirteen total Jins of pushing hands. There are not another thirteen postures. The five elements are advance, retreat backward, beware of the left, look to the right, and central equilibrium. They can be interpreted by dividing into internal and external. Those applied to the external are advance forward, retreat backward, beware of the left, look to the right, and central equilibrium. Those applied to the internal are attaching, connecting, adhering, following, and not lose contact and not resist.

十三勢者，按五行八卦原理，即推手之十三種總勁，非另有十三個姿勢。五行者，即進、退、顧、盼、定之謂。分為內外兩解。行於外者，即前進、後退、左顧、右盼、中定。行於內者，即粘、連、黏、隨、不丟頂。

Taijiquan was developed from the theory of Yin and Yang (Two Poles, 兩儀). From Yin and Yang, Four Phases (Si Xiang, 四象) were derived. From Four Phases, the Eight Trigrams (Bagua, 八卦) were initiated. The Eight Trigrams include Heaven (Qian, 乾), Earth (Kun, 坤), Water (Kan, 坎), Fire (Li, 離), Wind (Xun, 巽), Thunder (Zhen, 震), Lake (Dui, 兌), and Mountain (Gen, 艮) which correspond with the Taijiquan's eight basic moving patterns (i.e., basic Jins), Wardoff (Peng, 掤), Rollback (Lu, 擺), Press (Ji, 擠), Push (An, 按), Pluck (Cai, 採), Split (Lie, 挒), Elbow (Zhou, 肘), and Bump (Kao, 靠). In addition, Taijiquan also adopts the theory of the Five Elements (Wuxing, 五行). The Five Elements are Metal (Jin, 金),

Wood (Mu, 木), Water (Shui, 水), Fire (Huo, 火), and Earth (Tu, 土) which correspond with Taijiquan's five strategic steppings, Step Forward (Jin Bu, 進步), Step Backward (Tui Bu, 退步), Beware of the Left (Zuo Gu, 左顧), Look to the Right (You Pan, 右盼), and Central Equilibrium (Zhong Ding, 中定).

Based on these eight basic moving patterns, called Eight Doors (Ba Men, 八門), and five steppings, called Five Steppings (Wu Bu, 五步), Taijiquan techniques were developed. Therefore, Taijiquan is also called Thirteen Postures (Shi San Shi, 十三勢). From these thirteen basic movements, thirty-seven moving patterns were developed. Therefore, Taijiquan is also called Thirty-Seven Postures (San Shi Qi Shi, 三十七勢). That means Taijiquan is Thirteen Postures, also Thirty-Seven Postures.

When the theory of the Five Elements is applied to Taijiquan, externally it can be manifested into the five steppings. However, internally it contains the five important skills of attaching (Zhan, 粘), connecting (Lian, 連), adhering (Nian, 黏), following (Sui, 隨), and not lose contact and not resist (Bu Diu Bu Ding, 不丢不頂).

The eight trigrams can also be explained by dividing into internal and external. Those applying to the external are four directions and four corners. Those derived in the internal are Wardoff (Peng), Rollback (Lu), Press (Ji), Push (An), Pluck (Cai), Split (Lie), Elbow (Zhou), and Bump (Kao), eight techniques. What is manifested externally are postures and what is derived internally are Jins. The learners use the fist (Taiji sequence) as the body (i.e., main content) and the pushing hands as the applications. The classic says: "The root is at the feet, (Jin or movement is) generated from the legs, mastered (i.e., controlled) by the waist and manifested (i.e., expressed) at the fingers," is really the essential meaning of Taijiquan. The learners cannot be without awareness of it.

八卦者，亦分內外兩解。行於外者，即四正，四隅
。蘊於內者，即棚、攦、擠、按、採、挒、肘、靠
八法也。行於外者為勢，蘊於內者為勁。學者以拳
為體，以推手為用。經曰：〝其根在腳，發於腿，
主宰於腰，行於手指。〞實為太極拳之精義，學者
不可不留意焉。

When the theory of the Eight Trigrams is applied in the study of Taijiquan, externally it can be manifested to four sides and four corners as the eight directions of movement. Internally, its manifestations are Wardoff (Peng, 棚), Rollback (Lu, 攦), Press (Ji, 擠), Push (An, 按), Pluck (Cai, 採), Split (Lie, 挒), Elbow (Zhou, 肘), and Bump (Kao, 靠). In addition, when this theory is manifested externally (i.e., Yang), it is the postures or the external movements. When this theory is applied internally (i.e., Yin), it is using the mind to lead the Qi to derive the eight Jin patterns.

When you learn Taijiquan, first you learn a Taijiquan sequence. The Taijiquan sequence provides you with the main contents and the postures of the art. The form is like a book's table of contents. To learn how to apply these postures and movements into actual martial applications, you must first learn Taiji Pushing Hands. In fact, all of the movements or Jin manifestations are based on the theory stated in the ancient classic, *Taijiquan Treatise*, by Zhang, San-Feng (太極拳論 · 張三豐): "The root is at the feet, (Jin or movement is) generated from the legs, mastered (i.e., controlled) by the waist and manifested (i.e., expressed) at the fingers." If you can comprehend this sentence and apply it into action, you can move the entire body as a single unit. This means that you can move the entire body like a soft whip, infinitely smooth and unbroken.

The Detailed Interpretation of Five Elements

The five elements are metal, wood, water, fire, and earth. The Jins of five elements, says (i.e., are): attaching, connecting, adhering, following, and no losing and resisting. All of each Jin will be explained in detail next.

五行者，金、木、水、火、土也。五行之勁，曰粘
、連、黏、隨、不丟頂。茲將各勁詳解於後。

As explained earlier, the author of this poem believes that when the theory of the Five Elements is applied externally, it contains five strategic movements: Step Forward (Jin Bu, 進步), Step Backward (Tui Bu, 退步), Beware of the Left (Zuo Gu, 左顧), Look to the Right (You Pan, 右盼), and Central Equilibrium (Zhong Ding, 中定). When this theory is applied internally, it implies the five basic important Jin patterns. These Jins are: attaching (Zhan, 粘), connecting (Lian, 連), adhering (Nian, 黏), following (Sui, 隨), and no lose and no resist (Bu Diu Bu Ding, 不丟不頂). These five Jins will be explained next.

---

*(1). **Attaching:** Like the beginning of two objects connecting to one another. In Taijiquan terminology, this is called Jin. This Jin is not connecting (i.e., attaching) directly, but is generated indirectly. It contains the double meaning of both Jin and Yi. If in the middle of pushing hands or exchanging hands (i.e., sparring), the opponent's body is strong and large, Li (i.e., muscular force) and Qi are full and abundant, the stances are solid and firmed, it seems hard to make him move or shift his weighting center. However, if (I) use the attaching Jin, (it) can make him lose center automatically.*

五行要義詳解

Using Yi to probe (the opponent's Jin), make his Qi upraising and excited, and the whole spirit (i.e., whole mind) is focusing on the top. Then the body is heavy but the feet are light, his root will be broken automatically. This is caused because of the opponent's bounced Jin (i.e., natural reflex). I then follow the situation and release my hands, using the no losing and no resisting Jin, to lead the opponent suspended in the air (i.e., losing his root and center). This is the attaching Jin. The Jin is like attaching a ball, one touch and one lift, when apply it skillfully, the ball will not separate from hands. When attached, it immediately rises. This is what is called the attaching is yielding and the yielding is attaching.

〔一〕粘者。
如兩物互交粘之使起。在太極拳語中謂之勁。此勁
非直接粘起,實間接而生。含有勁意雙兼兩義。如
推手或交手時,對方體質強大,力氣充實,樁步穩
固,似難使其掀動,或移其重心,然以粘勁,能使
其自動失中。用意探之,使其氣騰,全神上住。則
體重而足輕,其根自斷。此即彼之反動力所致。吾
則順勢撒手,而以不丟不頂之勁,引彼懸空,是為
粘勁。夫勁如粘球,一撫一提之間,運用純熟,球
不離手,粘之即起。所謂粘即是走,走即是粘之謂
也。

The word of attaching (Zhan, 粘) is composed of two words, rice (Mi, 米) and occupying (Zhan, 占). In ancient times, glue was made from a starch such as rice or corn. When you use rice glue to occupy (i.e., stick) on some object it is called Zhan. It is just like when you stick a stamp with glue on an envelope. It is the same in Taijiquan. At the beginning of combat, your hands and your opponent's body are not yet connected. Therefore, you are unable to listen (i.e., feel), adhere, and follow. To connect, you must first attach. Attaching Jin is the first Jin in combat.

In order to attach, you must use your Yi (i.e., mind) and wait patiently for your opponent's attack in order to seize the advantageous situation and right timing. Then you can attach to the opponent. Often, you must initiate an insubstantial attack to trick the opponent into blocking, and from his block, you can attach to him. Direct attachment is rarely successful.

After the attachment, then you listen to (i.e., feel) and follow the opponent's force. Even after you have connected to the opponent, attaching Jin is still the most useful tool to defeat him. For example, if your opponent is big and strong, it is hard to destroy his balance and uproot him. You can use attaching Jin to influence his mind and make his Qi rise and become excited. In order to reach this goal, you must use your hand to attach to the opponent's center just like you are using your hand to attach to a ball (even if the hands have already connected to the opponent's body). When your opponent resists, you yield and let his power enter and when he retreats, again you attach to his center and push him off balance. If you can play these attaching and yielding tricks skillfully, you can influence the opponent's mind, make his spirit disturbed, and his Qi floating and excited. When this happens, you have controlled your opponent. The trick to success in this is that attaching (Yang) and yielding (Yin) must be used coordinatedly and skillfully.

What is the Yi, (it) means to the assumption (i.e., imagination). Using the theory of insubstantial and substantial, to attack the opponent with surprise when he is not prepared for it. Though the opponent's power is abundant (i.e., strong), he occupies the advantageous position, is not afraid of attack, and is not scared of a powerful opponent, still (he) is the most fearful of being baited and decoyed by his opponent. If I use the benefit to tempt him and make him give up his defense and replace it with offense, his power will be divided. Then, I attack the opponent's individual division. This is to decoy and then kill. This is also the opponent chooses to be defeated by himself. This is what is called "the Dao of attacking the places that are not defended and maintaining (i.e., keeping) the areas (i.e., conditions) where he is unable to attack." The learner must always try to comprehend this. After a long time, it (the above saying) will be verified automatically.

意者，設想之謂。以虛實之理，使敵出其不意，攻
其不備。對方雖實力充足，據險以守，不畏攻擊，
不畏力敵。然最忌誘敵，吾若以利誘之，使其棄守
為攻，實力分散，吾則分而擊之，是誘而殺之。亦
其自取敗亡。所謂攻其所不守，守其所不攻之道也
。學者務須時時體會，久而自驗。

The mind (i.e., Yi, 意) is the key to success. Use Yi to generate the insubstantial and substantial strategies. If your opponent is in the most advantageous situation, it is hard for you to find an opportunity to attack. In this case, you must use the attaching and yielding Jins to create a new situation which can confuse him and make him lose his confidence. Once your opponent is confused, then you will grasp the advantageous timing and situation to attack. The key strategy is to attack the places where he does not know how to defend himself and keep the opponent in the same weak conditions where he was weak (i.e., unable to attack). This means to attack the opponent's weak points and keep his weakness as it is.

––––––––––––––––––––

(2). **Connecting:** *(Means to) thread together, do not break, do not separate, connect and continuous, without stopping and endless, restless and ceaseless, is the connecting Jin.*

〔二〕連者。
貫也，不中斷，不脫離，接續聯綿，無停無止，無
息無休，是為連勁。

Connecting means to keep in touch with the opponent. It does not matter if the opponent moves or is still, my Jin remains connected with his body. This is called connecting Jin.

––––––––––––––––––––

(3). *Adhering: Means to attach and stick together. (When) the opponent advances, I retreat, (when) the opponent retreats, I advance. (When) the opponent is floating, I follow, (when) the opponent is sunken, I am loose. (He) cannot give up and separate, and cannot throw away and drop off. (It is) as attaching as sticking and do not lose and do not resist. This is called adhering Jin.*

〔三〕黏者。
粘貼之謂。彼進我退，彼退我進，彼浮我隨，彼沉
我鬆，丟之不開，投之不脫，如粘如貼，不丟不頂
，是謂之黏勁。

Once you have attached and connected with the opponent's body, your next task is to stick and adhere with him. In order to reach this goal, your skill of Listening Jin (Ting Jin, 聽勁)(i.e., feeling) must be very high. When your opponent advances, you follow, and when your opponent retreats, you advance. When his Jin is rising, you follow, and when his Jin is sunk, you keep yourself loose. If you resist, it will create a double weighting (Shuang Zhong, 雙重) (i.e., mutual resistance) situation and this will allow him to use his strong force to defeat you easily. If you stay loose, his sinking Jin will not find the root of sinking your Jin. In this case, he will lose the purpose of sinking.

When you adhere with your opponent, it is just like a piece of flypaper which sticks and adheres to his body. He cannot give it up or throw it away. This is the key to adhering Jin.

---

(4). *Following: (Means) to obey (i.e., follow the opponent's will). Slow and fast, (I) follow closely. Advance and retreat, I depend on (i.e., move along)(the opponent). Not controlling and not separating. Not prior and not after. Give up myself and follow the opponent is called following.*

〔四〕隨者。
從也。緩急相隨，進退相依，不即不離，不先不後
，舍己從人，是謂之隨。

In order to execute the Adhering Jin skillfully, you must also know how to follow the opponent's speed. It does not matter if he is advancing or retreating, follow his speed. Only then are you able to adhere with him. This means you give up your own opinion, and simply follow the opponent's idea and movement. This type of sur-render is quite difficult for many people. When it is achieved, you can use four ounces to lead one thousand pounds into emptiness (i.e., Neutralizing Jin)(Hua Jin, 化勁).

----

(5). **No Losing and No Resisting:** *Losing means separating. Resisting means to stiffen against. Do not separate, do not resist, do not be first, do not be behind. This is the origin of the five elements and the foundation of light and agile. This is the Jin of no losing and no resisting.*

〔五〕不丟頂。
丟者開也，頂者抵也。不脫離，不抵抗，不搶先，
不落後，五行之源，輕靈之本，是為不丟頂勁。

The last important key technique that corresponds to the five elements is the Jin of not losing contact and not resisting. This Jin corresponds to the earth. The earth is the neutral and center point of the five elements, and it coordinates and harmonizes the other four elements. This means that in order to attach, to connect, to adhere, and to follow, you must first know the skill of no losing and no resist-ing. Only then can you execute the other four skills with agility.

The Secrets of Eight Techniques

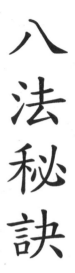

How do we explain the Wardoff Jin (Peng Jin)? Like the water is carrying a moving boat. First solidify (i.e., fill up) the Qi in the Lower Dan Tian. Next, the head must be suspended upward. The springing force is originated from the entire body. Opening and closing have their definite timing. It does not matter (if the coming force) is a thousand pounds of weight, (it) is not hard to make (the opponent) float (i.e., uprooted).

棚勁義何解，如水負行舟。先實丹田氣，次要頂頭懸。
全體彈簧力，開合一定間。任有千斤重，飄浮亦不難。

According to the Eight Trigrams, Wardoff Jin (Peng Jin, 棚勁) is an extreme Yang Jin which belongs to Heaven (☰)(Qian, 乾). This implies that it is strong and powerful. Although it is powerful enough to carry a boat like water, it can flow and move smoothly, freely, and with ultimate fluidity. In pushing hands, Wardoff Jin can not only be used for offense but also for defense. When it is used for defense, it is like water slipping under the prow of a boat, carrying it smoothly, swiftly and effortlessly. In a similar way the opponent's power is "carried" and lead into emptiness. Peng Jin is the first and the most important Jin pattern in Taijiquan. It is a crucial topic to understand, and the ability to manifest the Jin is critical to progress in the art.

In order to manifest strong power, you must first learn how to fill up the Qi in the Lower Dan Tian. Qi is the energy that allows the physical body to manifest its power. When the Dan Tian Qi is full, the power can be strong. Not only that, the spirit of vitality must be high. In order to raise up this spirit, the head must be upright. Once you have a strong Qi flow to support the physical body and a high spirit, you must then learn how to manifest the power like a spring from any point in the body. In addition, to make the Jin's manifestation effective, when you apply Wardoff Jin, the timing and the opportunity must be accurate. Once you can reliably execute the above elements, even if your opponent's force is a thousand pounds, you can neutralize it and make him uprooted.

How do we explain the Rollback Jin (Lu Jin)? To lead and make (the opponent's force) forward. Follow the coming force and be light and agile without losing and resisting. (When the coming) force ends, it will enter the emptiness naturally. Throw or attack (the opponent) following the natural situation (i.e., opportunity). (My) weight center should be maintained and do not let the opponent take the opportunity.

攦勁義何解，引導使之前。順其來時力，輕靈不丟頂。
力盡自然空，丟擊任自然。重心自維持，莫被他人乘。

According to the Eight Trigrams, Rollback Jin (Lu Jin, 攦勁) is an extremely Yin Jin that belongs to the Earth (☷)(Kun, 坤). This implies that it is used mainly defensively, commonly to lead and neutralize the opponent's incoming force into emptiness.

The first step in applying Rollback Jin is to yield and lead the opponent's force forward, then to re-direct it to the sides and finally lead it into emptiness. In order to make Rollback Jin effective, you must first know the crucial key to no losing and no resisting. Furthermore, you must always maintain your center. If you do not have a firm center, you will not have firm balance to neutralize the incoming force effectively. This will also provide your opponent with an opportunity to attack you with his elbow or bump you off balance with his shoulder or body.

How do we explain the Press Jin (Ji Jin)? When applying, use both sides. (When apply) directly, the mind is pure and simple. Meet and combine are (occurring) in

a single movement. (When apply) indirectly to gener-
ate the rebounding force, it is like a ball's rebound after
hitting the wall. It is also like throwing a coin to hit a
drum, (it) is bouncing and the sound is clear.

擠勁義何解，用時用兩方。直接單純意，迎合一動中。
間接反應力，如球撞壁還。又如錢投鼓，躍然聲鏗鏘。

The meaning of Ji (擠) in Chinese is to squeeze or to press against. When it is used to squeeze, the force is from both sides towards the center. For example, when your opponent pushes your chest with both of his hands, you may simply use both of your hands to squeeze his elbows toward the center and downward to neutralize his attack. The purpose of this kind of application is straightforward, and therefore the "mind" is very simple. However, if you use the press to generate a press Jin, the force is a spring-like bouncing power. When the Jin is emitted, it is clean and clear.

How do we explain the Pushing Jin (An Jin)? Its appli-
cations are like the water's moving. The hardness is
hidden within the softness. The turbulence is so urgent
that its coming force is hard to resist. When encounter-
ing the high (situation), then the tide is high. When
encountering the low situation, then the tide is diving
downward. The waves have the up and down motions,
and there are no holes that cannot be entered.

按勁義何解，運用似水行。柔中寓剛強，急流勢難當。
遇高則澎滿，逢窪向下潛。波浪有起伏，有孔無不入。

The word An (按) is constructed from two words, hand (Shou, 扌) and peace (An, 安). This implies that the technique of An is to use the hand(s) to make peace (i.e., calm down). The action of An is to calm down the incoming force by settling the wrist (Zuo Wan, 坐腕). For example, if your opponent pushes your chest with both of his hands, you may simply press or push down his two shoulders with your two hands to immobilize his intention. Naturally, An can be applied upward, downward, or any direction. Therefore, when it is applied, it is like water which can flow anywhere. However, hidden within this soft flowing is a hardness in action when the wrist is settling. This action can be used to strike the cavities or vital areas.

How do we explain the Pluck Jin (Cai Jin)? It is like using a gauge to test the balance. It does not matter how the opponent's force is huge or slender, after gauging then know the (coming force) is light or heavy. The turning and shifting is only four ounces, even (the coming force) is a thousand pounds, (I) can still (to turn and shift it). If asked the reason behind it, it is the application of torque (i.e., leverage).

採勁義何解，如權之引衡。任你力巨細，權後知輕重。
轉移祇四兩，千斤亦可乎。若問理何在，幹捍之作用。

Pluck (Cai, 採) is commonly used to control the opponent's elbows and wrists. Pluck is not a grabbing. Because when you grab, you will be tense. When you pluck, you are using your hands (thumb and index finger or thumb and middle finger) to pluck the opponent's wrist or elbow and lead the incoming force downward, upward, or to the side. When you use pluck, you must use it at the right moment. First, you must be able to gauge the opponent's power and how well he can maintain his center and balance. Once you can shift his center and balance, with the assistance of pluck, you can even use just four ounces to neutralize one thousand pounds. All success in this depends on how you make your opponent lose his balance.

How do we explain the Split Jin (Lie Jin)? Spinning like a flying wheel. (When) there is an object thrown on it, (it will be) thrown more than ten feet away. Don't you see the whirlpool, its turning waves are like the spi-

*ral lines. When a falling leave lands on it, (the leave)
will sink and perish hastily.*

捌勁義何解，旋轉若飛輪。投物於其上，脫然擲丈尋。
君不見漩渦，捲浪若螺紋。落葉墮其上，倐爾便沉淪。

Split (Lie, 捌) is to generate a spinning force from the body to
either strike or bounce the opponent off balance. Normally, Split
Jin is forward and to the side. It is like a double whirlpool or like a
double helix, or like two tornados going in opposite directions in an
hourglass shape. The energy looks like an hourglass. The whirlpool
spins and draws everything down into it. Powerful whirlpools are
called maelstroms or vortices.

---

*How do we explain the Elbow Jin (Zhou Jin)? Its meth-
ods have five possibilities. Yin and Yang are divided
into up and down, the insubstantial and substantial
must be discriminated clearly. The continuous linking
attacking forces are hard to defeat. When the flower
blooming strikes (i.e., circle the forearm for a fist strike),
it is even more fierce. (When) the six Jins are blended
and threaded together, the unlimited applications will
begin.*

肘勁義何解，方法有五行。陰陽分上下，虛實須辨清。
連環勢莫擋，開花捶更凶。六勁融通後，運用始無窮。

There are five possibilities in the application of Elbow Jin. Elbow
Jin (Zhou Jin, 肘勁) can be moved up and down as Yin or Yang. It
can also be used as an insubstantial and substantial strategy. In addition, Elbow Jins can be used continuously (i.e., one after another).
Together with these five possible manifestations of Jin, if you also
know how to use the Jin of circling fist, then the applications of
Elbow Jin can be unlimited. It is very important to understand that
when the Elbow Jin is used, one must beware if the opponent knows
how to use pluck to control the elbow and direct the Jin away or lead

you into an awkward situation. However, if you know how to use circling fist Jin (i.e., flower blooming), you can strike the opponent's face whenever your elbow is plucked.

How do we explain the Bump Jin (Kao Jin)? Its techniques are divided into using the shoulders or back. Diagonal flying uses the shoulder and within the (application of) shoulder, there is also a back. Once gaining the advantageous position, (bump the opponent) with a deafening sound like a pounding pestle. Be careful to keep the weighting center, (if) losing it, the effort will be in vain.

靠勁義何解，其法分肩背。斜飛勢用肩，肩中還有背。
一旦得機勢，轟然如搗碓。仔細維重心，失中徒無功。

Kao (靠) means to bump the opponent off balance. There are many places in your body that can be used to bump the opponent, such as the shoulders, back, hips, thighs, chest, or even the knees. However, in Taijiquan pushing hands, the shoulder and the back are the places most commonly used. For example, in the posture of diagonal flying, the shoulder is often used to bump the opponent. However, if the opponent is very close, the back can also be used effectively. When you apply bump Jin, the timing and situation must be appropriate. Once you grasp that you are in an advantageous situation, do not hesitate to generate a strong bumping force to bump the opponent off balance. There must be no hesitation, however, and your realization and action must be almost unconscious and as one. Whenever you apply bump Jin, you must first have a firm root, center, and balance. Otherwise, the bump Jin will not be effective. Furthermore, the rebounded Jin from the opponent can also bump you off balance.

The Interpretation of Slow and Without Force

慢與不用力之解釋

Taijiquan is slow and without force, many of the learners doubt about it (i.e., its martial usage). Perhaps it is said that it cannot be applied (in fighting) and can only be used for body training (i.e., health). However, the Dao of training fist (i.e., martial arts) should first study and research the learning theory. After learning the theory and understanding it clearly, then learn the techniques. The techniques must be mastered and refined, then they can be useful. Not the fist techniques cannot be used, it is because the Gongfu (of training) has not yet been achieved. It is like refining steel. From raw iron (i.e., iron ore) refined into ripe iron, from ripe iron then refined into pure steel. Without long time of refining, the goal cannot be achieved.

太極拳慢而無力，學者多懷疑之。或謂不能應用，
徒能鍛練身體。蓋練拳之道，首宜研究學理。學理
瞭然，再學方法。方法精熟，始能應用。非拳術之
不能應用，實功夫之尚未練到耳。如鍊鋼然。由生
鐵，而鍊成熟鐵。由熟鐵，而鍊成純鋼。非經過長
時間之火候不為功。

Many Taijiquan practitioners doubt if Taijiquan can be used as a martial art. The reason for this is that at the beginning, Taijiquan training emphasizes softness, relaxation, and not using any muscular power. However, if a Taijiquan practitioner understands the Taijiquan training theory clearly, he will see that when Taijiquan is trained to a high level, with internal mind and Qi training, it can be performed slow or fast. It can also be soft like cotton or hard like steel. Therefore, in order to reach a deep profound level of Taijiquan training, the first task is to study the theory and understand it clearly.

Next, you must train hard and apply the theory into the action. If you do not train correctly (i.e., because you do not understand the theory) and do not practice hard (i.e., Gongfu), you will not be able to use Taijiquan as a martial art. This passage concludes that understanding the theory and training intelligently are the two keys to reach proficient levels of the Taijiquan art.

The reason that Taijiquan is achieved from slow (movements) is because during the practice, (it) follows the nature (way). (It) does not emphasize strength but focuses on (the training of) using the Yi (i.e., wisdom mind). (If) use (only) muscular strength, then clumsy. (If) use (only) Qi, then stagnant. Therefore, the most important (things) in the training are to sink the Qi (to the Lower Dan Tian) and loosen the muscular power. Taijiquan uses calmness to subdue the movement, uses softness to control the hardness. Generate having (i.e., something) from nothingness. Having as if not having, substantial as if insubstantial. When the adverse comes, (I) follow

a 夫太極拳之所以由慢而成者，其練習時間，純任自 e
b 然。不尚力氣，而尚用意。用力則笨，用氣則滯。 !
是以沉氣鬆力為要。太極拳，以靜制動，以柔制剛
，無中生有。有若無，實若虛。逆來順受，不丟不
頂。均係虛實之變化也。

Why is Taijiquan practiced with slow motion? The answer is because it emphasizes the Yi (意)(i.e., wisdom mind). Use the Yi to lead the Qi and then manifest it into Jins. In order to have effective Jin manifestation, the Qi must be abundant and sunk. In order to circulate the Qi in the body smoothly, freely, and naturally, the body must be loose and relaxed. Once you can do this, your feeling and sensitivity will be higher than your opponent's. When this happens, you can govern the entire battle situation. Use calmness to defend against movement, use softness to defeat hardness, and also be able to change your strategy skillfully. In this case, your opponent will not be able to figure out your insubstantial and substantial. However, to reach this skillful level, you must invest great effort and time.

――――――――――――――

Slow, means unhasting. Slow, it (i.e., the mind) can be calm. Calm, it (i.e., the Qi) can be kept (at the center). (When) it (i.e., Qi) can be kept (at the center), it means steady. This is the Xin (i.e., emotional mind) and Qi's central equilibrium. The Xin is steady and then can be calm. When calm, then the spirit can be peaceful. When the spirit is peaceful, the Qi can be sunk. When the Qi is sunk, then the spirit of vitality can be gathered. Then (you) can gather the essence and meet the spirit (i.e., concentrate) and the sole Qi can thread through (the entire body). Slow originated from the refined Xin (i.e., cautiousness). When the Xin is coarse (i.e., careless) then impatient, impatient, then the Qi is floating. When Qi is floating and not sinking, then the Xin is impatient and not calm. Not sinking and not calm, the Xin can not be kept (at the center), then the sickness of random and confusion is generated.

慢者，緩也。慢所以靜，靜所以守，守之謂定。此
即心氣之中定也。心定而後靜，靜而後神安，神安
而後氣沉，氣沉而後精神團聚，乃能聚精會神，一
氣貫通。慢由心細，心細則神清，神清則氣爽，乃
無氣滯之弊。快由於心粗，心粗由於急，急則氣浮
，氣浮不沉，心急不靜。不沉不靜，心無所守，則
散亂之病生。

The reason for being slow is that, when you move slowly, you can become calm. When you are calm, then you can keep your Xin (i.e., emotional mind) and Qi at their centers. In this case, your mind and body will be peaceful and steady. When this happens, you are sensitive and the response to the opponent's intention will be clear and wise. This is the central equilibrium of the Xin and

Qi. Therefore, calmness is the crucial key to a deep and profound sensitivity and presence.

———————

Insubstantial and agility two words, (we) cannot ask more (than these two). Using the calmness to subdue the movement and using the softness to defeat the hardness are all possible due to the touching and feeling. Therefore, the fist postures are used to train the physical and mental bodies as the main object (i.e., main content). Gongfu (i.e., the achievement) is originated from pushing hands and is the applications. At the beginning stage of pushing hands, (you) should focus on the training of touching and feeling. The body has been touched, the mind (immediately) feels. The response is refined and detailed and the applications are unlimited. Therefore, (you) can know yourself and (your) opponent. Its taste (i.e., the essence of the art) can only be obtained from the mind's comprehension and spiritual gathering (i.e., concentration). It cannot be described with the pen. Its variations are unlimited, all from the sensitivity of feeling. Therefore, (you) can know the opponent's insubstantial and substantial and conveniently allow (you) to apply (the techniques) as wished. This is the meaning of slow and not using the force.

虛靈二字，更無由求。以靜制動，以柔剋剛者，由於感覺使然。故拳架係鍛練身心以為體。功夫出自推手而為用。推手之初步，專在摩練感覺。身有所感，心有所覺。感應精微，致用無窮。故能知己知彼。其滋味則心領神會，非筆墨所能形容。其變化之無窮，皆由感覺之靈敏。故能知其虛實，而便利從心。此慢與不用力之義也。

When you are insubstantial, you are defensive and in ready position for any action or reaction. In this case, your mind must be calm so you can use the calmness to handle your opponent's movement. In addition, you must be agile. In order to be agile, your feeling (i.e., Listening Jin) must be high, your contact with the opponent must be light. When this happens, you can be agile.

If you practice Taijiquan only for solo forms, what you will learn will be only postures and movements. If you wish to apply the techniques in the martial arts, you must practice pushing hands. From pushing hands, you learn the feeling (i.e., Listening Jin). The more sensitive your feeling, the better your mind can understand the opponent's intention. Once you have reached a high level of sensitivity, you can execute your insubstantial and substantial strategies efficiently and effectively.

中
定

Central Equilibrium

Before the action of extending, bending, opening, and closing is called center. Extremely quiet (i.e., calm) without movement is called steady (i.e., equilibrium, balanced, and rooted). The heart (i.e., emotional mind) and the Qi are clean and harmonious, the spirit of vitality reaches the top (of the head), no tilting no leaning, is the Qi of central equilibrium. It is also the root of the Dao (i.e., Taijiquan).

伸屈開合之未發謂之中。寂然不動謂之定，心氣清
和，精神貫頂，不偏不倚，是為中定之氣，亦道之
本也。

When your mind is at the center of gravity (i.e., Real Dan Tian, 真丹田), you are in the Wuji (無極) state. In this state, you do not have any intent; simply keep your physical center and mental center centered. This state is called the central state. Once you are in this central state, keep your mind calm, sink your Qi to the Lower Dan Tian, and lead the Qi to the top of your head. The sinking downward of the Qi is to build up the root, and the leading of the Qi upward is to raise up the spirit of vitality. When you have firm rooting and a high spirit, you can act with balance. In this case, you will also have equilibrium. Central equilibrium belongs to the earth in the five elements. All of the relaxed Taijiquan movements build on central equilibrium. Once you have lost it, you will be tensed and uprooted.

Insubstantiality Leading the Head Upward

虛領頂勁

The Jin of leading upward means the head is suspended from above. The head is upward and upright, the abdomen is relaxed and clean internally. The Qi is sinking to the (Lower) Dan Tian, the spirit of vitality reaches the top (of the head). It is just like the toy tumbler. The top is light and the low is sunk. It is also like the floating buoy, floating and swaying around will not sink. It can be sung as: "The spirit is clean (i.e., clear) and the Qi is sinking and follow the natural (way), floating, swaying and boring in the wave. It does not matter how (strong) the wind and wave strike, the top is light and the bottom is sunk without turning upside down.

頂勁者，即頂頭懸。頭頂正直，腹內鬆淨，氣沉丹田，精神貫頂，如不倒翁，上輕下沉。又如水中浮漂，漂然不沒之意。歌曰：「神清氣沉任自然，漂漂盪盪浪裡攢。憑你風浪來推打，上輕下沉不倒顛。」

An insubstantial energy leads the head upward. This means to raise up the spirit of vitality. In order to raise up the spirit, the Qi must also be always sinking downward to the Lower Dan Tian. To have abundant Qi storage in the Lower Dan Tian, the abdominal area must be relaxed. When this happens, you will have a firm root while the head is always kept upright. With a loose waist, you can neutralize the incoming force and protect your center and balance.

27

感覺 Feeling and Sensing

When the body has a touch, the heart (i.e., mind) has the feeling. Whenever there is a touch, there must be a response. All of the movements and calmness are the touches, therefore they must also have responses. After responses, then again there are touches. After touches, again there must be responses. Therefore, they are repeatedly producing each other without stop. The theory of touching and responding is very refined and profound until (they) can be applied (in situations). At the beginning of (learning) pushing hands, (you) should be focusing on the (training of) touching and feeling. (When) the touching and feeling are sensitive and acute, then the variations will be refined and detailed and therefore, (the applications) can be unlimited.

身有所感，心有所覺，有感必有應。一切動靜皆為
感，感則必有應，所應復為感，所感復有應，所以
互生不已。感通之理，精義入微，以致用也。推手
初步，專在摩練感覺。感覺靈敏，則變化精微，所
以無窮也。

In the general combat situation, the most important factor for winning is reaction. When your eyes see the opponent's action (even a slight movement), immediately your mind is aware of it and responds to it. Your body must also react quickly to the mind's decision. All of these corresponding actions are called reaction.

However, in Taijiquan pushing hands or even combat situations, after the interception (i.e., attachment) of the opponent's attack, you immediately stick and adhere with the opponent. Not stick to, as this implies an exertion or effort, but stick and adhere with him, listening and responding to the movements you sense from his center. This is a short range fighting situation. When this happens, the feeling of the skin in your body (i.e., Listening Jin) is extremely important. The more sensitive your skin is, the more you can feel and sense the opponent's intention. Therefore, this feeling of sensitivity is a most important language that allows you to communicate with your opponent. Once you have sensitive feeling and sensing, then you must ponder how the mind can correspond with this feeling. This is the step of awareness.

After it has received the message of the feeling, the mind must immediately respond and react. This means you are answering the opponent's attack. Naturally, in order to protect himself, your opponent will again answer back. This questioning and answering process repeats continuously until one side has won. From this you can see that success depends on the feeling (i.e., Listening Jin). This means that at the beginning of pushing hands practice, you should pay attention to this feeling. Only after you have established a sensitive feeling are you able to understand the Jin (i.e., Understanding Jin). Only after you understand the Jin, can you reply to the opponent's action precisely with the most advantageous timing and opportunity.

聽勁 Listening Jin

Listening means to gauge. That means to gauge the light or heavy (of the coming Jin). In pushing hands, it means to detect the enemy's conditions. Listening (i.e., feel) in the heart, condensed (i.e., pay attention) in the ears, transport with Qi and apply it at the hands. It is what is called: "Use the Xin (i.e., emotional mind) to mobilize the Yi (i.e., wisdom mind), use the Yi to move the Qi, and use the Qi to manifest the body. Listening (first) and then emitting. The Listening Jin must be accurate and sensitively acute. Follow his (i.e., the opponent's) extending, and ensue his bending, then (you) can advance and retreat as wish.

聽之謂權，即權其輕重也。在推手為偵察敵情。聽
之於心，凝之於耳，行之於氣，運之於手。所謂以
心行意，以意行氣，以氣運身，聽而後發。聽勁要
準確靈敏，隨其伸，就其屈，乃能進退自如。

Listening in Taijiquan pushing hands and sparring means the feeling of the skin. When this level goes beyond feeling, it is the sense of the opponent's intention. After listening, you immediately gauge the opponent's intention, his power, and his capability. From the gauging, you can understand the situation in your heart. Therefore, listening (i.e., feeling) is the first contact with the opponent. It is the detector which helps the mind collect the information.

After listening, the Xin (心)(i.e., emotional mind) immediately responds. From the Xin, the message passes to the Yi (意)(i.e., wisdom mind). In order to make your alertness reach a high level, not only is your skin's feeling important, your eyes' sensitivity and your ears' listening are also important. In fact, you are using all of the sensing organs to detect the opponent's action. Once the Yi has decided on a responsive action, immediately the Yi leads the Qi to the physical body for manifestation of power. If you do not carefully listen in the first place, and make a decision without knowing the opponent's situation, you will be placed in a disadvantageous position.

From this, you can tell that listening Jin is very important. It must be accurate and fast. Without correct information, your response to the opponent's action will naturally be unpredictable and often wrong. After listening, then you can follow the opponent and lead the incoming force into emptiness (Hua Jin, 化勁)(i.e., Neutralization Jin). You will also be able to advance and retreat as you wish.

問答 Questions and Answers

(When) I ask question, the opponent will respond with the answer. One questions and one answers, then movements and stillness are generated. Once there are the movements and calmness, the insubstantial and substantial can be discriminated clearly. In pushing hands, (first) use the Yi to probe, use the Jin to ask, once receiving the response, again listen (i.e., feel) his insubstantial and substantial. If (I) ask and without any response, then (I) can advance and attack. (However), if there is a response, then (I) must listen the slow and fast of his movements and stillness, and also the direction of his advancing and retreating, then (I) am able to discriminate his insubstantial and substantial.

我有所問，彼有所答。一問一答，則生動靜。既有
動靜，虛實分明。在推手則以意探之。以勁問之。
俟其答覆，再聽其虛實。若問而不答，則可進而擊
之。若有所答，則須聽其動靜之緩急，及進退之方
向，始能辨其虛實也。

Questioning and answering means to exchange techniques with the opponent. When I am questioning, that means I am detecting and initiating an action. Once the action is initiated, I must be careful and see if there is an answer. If there is no answer, that means the opponent's listening (i.e., feeling) is not sensitive enough to my attack. Naturally, I should continue my attack.

However, once you have initiated a question and your opponent responds with an answer, then the mutual exchanges of the techniques will be starting. When this happens, you must be careful to distinguish the opponent's insubstantial and substantial clearly. Do not enter his trap and place yourself into a disadvantageous position.

Therefore, you must constantly use your Yi (i.e., wisdom mind) to gauge the situation, and then use the Jin to test the opponent. Once you have the answer, you immediately discriminate his insubstantial and substantial. In addition, you must also understand the speed of his Jin and how he directs his power toward you. Once you can detect and feel all of this, you will be capable of discriminating the insubstantial and substantial.

虛實 Insubstantial and Substantial

(When using) soldiers, do not detest applying the deceits. (or Trickery is not vice in military operations.) This is to use guile to defeat the opponent. The plot (or trick) is what is called the insubstantial and substantial. It is the same in the applications of Fist Techniques (i.e., martial techniques). The postures, the movements, the usage of the mind, and applications of the Jin all have insubstantial and substantial. (You should) know the insubstantial and substantial and be good at using them. Though (it looks like) insubstantial, it is substantial and though (it acts like) substantial, it is insubstantial. Use (my) substantial to attack the (opponent's) insubstantial and avoid the (opponent's) substantial and attack his insubstantial. Pointing up but striking low, (making) noise at the east but striking at the west, or first (my Jin) is heavy and then light, or first is light and then heavy. Hidden and apparent are not normal (i.e., regular). Sinking and floating are not regular. Make the opponent not know my insubstantial and substantial and I am always probing the opponent's insubstantial and substantial. (If) the opponent's (Jin) is substantial, then (I) evade and (if) the opponent's (Jin) is insubstantial, then (I) attack. Vary (my strategy) following the situation. Listen to his Jin, observe his movements, gain the opportunity and attack his void. If a doctor diagnoses a patient and applies the herbs, first, (he) must feel the patient's pulse, observe his color (of the face), and investigate his sound, and ask his conditions. Therefore, it is said: "Insubstantial and substantial must be discriminated clearly. Each place has each place's insubstantial and substantial.

Everywhere are all the same having insubstantial and substantial.

兵不厭詐，以計勝人也。計者，虛實之謂。拳術亦
然。姿勢，動作、用意、運勁各有虛實。知虛實而
善利用。雖虛為實，雖實猶虛。以實擊虛，避實擊
虛。指上打下，聲東擊西。或先重而後輕，或先輕
而後重。隱現無常，沉浮不定。使敵不知吾之虛實
，而吾處處求敵之虛實。彼實則避之，彼虛則擊之
。隨機應變。聽其勁，觀其動，得其機，攻其勢。
如醫者視病而投藥，必先診其脈，觀其色，察其聲
，問其症。故曰：〝虛實宜分清楚。一處有一處虛
實。處處總此一虛實也。〞

Insubstantial and substantial action is a strategy and is a military trick commonly used to confuse the opponent. It is the same in combat situations in Taijiquan. All success in executing the plot depends on how well you understand your opponent. Therefore, you must probe his situation to become aware of his insubstantial and substantial, and at the same time vary your strategy accordingly. The more you can discriminate the opponent's insubstantial and substantial, the better you can execute your insubstantial and substantial strategy.

量
敵

Gauging the Opponent

The military tactics say: "knowing myself and knowing the opponent, hundred battles, hundred victories." Therefore, at the beginning of gathering the army and the journey for an attack, always first investigate ourselves and gauge the opponent (i.e., know the opponent), and evaluate the possibility of winning and losing. This saying is really sincerely truthful. The tricky (key) of winning or losing depends on if (I) know or do not know (the opponent). Though the fist (i.e., martial art) is a small Dao (i.e., fighting art), its theory remains the same. Using my short (i.e., faults, the skills I am not good at) against the opponent's long (i.e., expertise) means losing the tactics. Using my long (i.e., expertise) to defeat the opponent's short, means to have gained the tactics. The Dao of winning victory is decided in the gaining or losing. Therefore, gauging the opponent is the most important (in a battle).

兵法云：〝知己知彼，百戰百勝。〞是故整軍行旅
之初，常先審己量敵，而計其勝負之情也。誠哉斯
言。勝負之機，在知與不知耳。拳雖小道，其理亦
然。以己之短，當人之長，謂之失計。以己之長，
當人之短，謂之得計。取勝之道，在得失之間。故
量敵最關重要也。

The first sentence of this paragraph is from Sun Wu's book of military tactics. Sun Wu (孫武), also known as Sun Zi (Mister Sun, 子), (and in the West as Sun Tzu), was a very famous strategist who lived around 557 B.C. His book *Sun Zi's Fighting Strategies* (*Sun Zi Bing Fa*, 孫子兵法)(often translated *"The Art of War"*) has been studied by Chinese soldiers for centuries, and has become required reading in most military schools throughout the world. Although phrased

36

in terms of battles and troop movements, the book applies equally well to individual conflicts.

In order to pursue victory, you must know your opponent and yourself. Therefore, the first step in pushing hands competition, as in battle, is to probe or to investigate the opponent's capability and his expertise. Only after you have some intelligence on your opponent and your relative capabilities can you set up an effective strategy to win the battle.

In Taijiquan, in order to know your opponent, the first step is to build up high sensitivity in Listening Jin. The purpose of Listening Jin (Ting Jin, 聽勁)(i.e., feeling and sensing) is to collect information. Then, you must understand the opponent's intention. This is called Understanding Jin (Dong Jin, 懂勁). After you have gone through these two processes, you can then set up an effective fighting strategy to win the battle. To gauge the opponent means to listen and to understand the opponent's intention and capability.

What is called question and answer in Taijiquan is to investigate the opponent's movement and calmness. Its goal is to listen (for) the direction and heavy center (i.e., the origin or the root) of his Jin. This means to probe the opponent's situation. It is what is called to gauge the opponent. Before the opponent and I engage the battle, I should use the calmness to wait for (his) movements, and use the ease to wait for the labor without any formed opinion (i.e., guessing). The opponent does not move, I do not move. The opponent slightly moves, I move first. The most precious moment is the instant of mutual exchange between the opponent and I, when (if I) know the opponent's insubstantial and substantial, I can deal with it. All of these (possibilities) are originated from (the) feeling of Listening Jin, insubstantial and substantial, question and answer, and gauging the opponent. The practitioner should pay attention to put all the effort in these.

太極拳之所謂問答，即問其動靜。目的在聽其勁之
方向與重心，即偵察敵情之意，所謂量敵也。彼我
在未進行攻擊以前，吾應以靜待動，以逸待勞，毫
無成見。彼未動，我不動，彼微動，我先動。貴在
彼我相交一動之間，即知其虛實而應付之。此均由
於感覺。聽勁、虛實、問答、量敵而來。學者應注
意致力焉。

In order to understand your opponent, you must first give your opponent a few tests. From these tests, you can understand his capability and expertise. To reach this goal, normally you must initiate a few testing attacks—these attacks are called questions. After you have initiated a question, you will wait for the answer. That means waiting for your opponent's response to your attack. From the exchange of questioning and answering, you can see your opponent's talent and fighting capability. This step is called gauging the opponent.

After knowing your opponent, you then wait for his action patiently. Use defensive as offensive strategy. Use a calm mind to wait for his first movement. Take ease and do not hurry. Do not guess the opponent's intention and action. Simply keep calm and wait. When he does not move, you will not move. Once he just starts to initiate an attack, you move first. This is because when he has just slightly moved to initiate an attack, his mind is on the offense and not in defensive alertness. If you can attack at this time, you can catch the best timing for your attack.

All of this happens quickly, and winning or not is decided in an instant. All of the possibilities for reaching this goal depend on the capability of your Listening Jin, your knowledge of your opponent through the questioning and answering process, and how well you can understand your opponent's insubstantial and substantial.

Knowing the Opportunity

知機

What is the opportunity? It has no discrimination of Yin and Yang, (and it is) nothingness, remote and vague. When it is said the opportunity, it means knowing the opportunity before its happening. It has no sound, no smelling, no shape, and no image. When it is applied, there is no movement and calmness, and the postures (i.e., situation) are not yet formed. Therefore, there is no opportunity. Those people who have reached a high level of Gongfu are all able to know the opportunity, and can create the situation. It is what is called able to create having (opportunity) from nothing, able to catch the opportunity and engage the action. Those who are low (in Gongfu), do not know the opportunity and therefore cannot catch the advantage. It is what is called: "Three levels of achievement in our Dao (i.e., Taijiquan): those who know and are aware of prior (opportunity), those who know and are aware of latter (opportunity), those who do not know and are not aware of any (opportunity)." Those who belong to our gate (i.e., our style, meaning Wu style), once have experienced the pushing hands (training) will comprehend (the above saying) automatically. Then it is not necessary to combat for winning and losing to see who is higher or lower (in skill) between the opponent and I.

機者，陰陽未分，虛無緲茫。謂之機，先機之謂也
。即是無聲無臭，無形無象。在應用時，是未有動
靜，未成姿勢，是無機會也。工夫高者，皆能知機
，能造勢。所謂無中生有，乘機而動。下者，不知
機，故不得勢。所謂先知先覺，後知後覺，不知不
覺，此為吾道之三大境界。凡屬吾門，一經推手，
自然領會，彼我之高下，無須相角勝負。

The opportunity itself does not have Yin or Yang, nor can it be seen. This is because normally, if there is no obvious appearance or manifestation of the opponent's intention, you cannot see the opportunity. Therefore, there is no opportunity for you to take an advantageous action. However, if your skill is high and developed, you can know the opponent clearly and control the situation. When this happens, you can create the opportunity and advantageous situation. In this case, you have transformed a no opportunity situation into a situation with opportunity. Those martial artists with lower level skill will not be able to create opportunity and catch the advantageous situation. Therefore, skill can be divided into three levels. The highest contains those who know the opponent and can feel the opponent's intention and control the situation. The second level of skill is comprised of those who have to wait after the opponent has manifested his intention and then react. The lowest level consists of those who do not understand or are not even aware the opportunity at all. Because of this, normally after the first few technique exchanges, you can already know who is going to win a battle.

It is just like playing chess. Those who have achieved the high level, whenever they place a piece, there is an intention. The eyes (i.e., vision) see far and never lose the target when attacking. All the pieces they place are linked together and the Qi (i.e., life force) is connected. When this advantageous situation has been taken, winning or losing (i.e., victory) has already been decided. Those who have achieved low level, the vision is shallow and near, the heart (i.e., mind) does not have grown bamboo (i.e., confidence). Therefore, they cannot catch the advantageous situation and (are) controlled by the opponent. (When this happens), they will not have leisure time to take care of themselves (i.e., protect themselves). Its losing has already been known. It is the same theory in pushing hands. Those who have achieved a high level, the heart (i.e., mind) and the Qi are sunken and calm, the postures are greatly elegant (i.e., comfortable and sure), can follow the adverse (situation), and apply (the skills) as they wish. Those who have reached only the low level, there is no door when advance, there is no escape when retreat. (They) are unable to attack and have no (effective) techniques to defend (themselves). This is the difference of knowing the opportunity and not knowing the opportunity.

譬如圍棋，高者每下一子，皆有用意，眼光遠大，
著不虛發，氣俱聯貫，而占局勢，其勝負之情已定
。下者，眼光淺近，心無成竹，不得先手，隨人擺
脫，而自顧不暇，其必敗也已知。推手之理亦然。
高者，心氣沉靜，姿態大雅，逆來順受，運用自如
。下者，進則無門，退則無路，攻之不可，守之無
術。此即知機與不知機之分耳。

All of the theories in creating and grasping the advantageous opportunity in pushing hands are analogous to the principles of chess. Those who have reached a high level can create different advantageous situations that all link with and support each other. When this happens, they can control the entire situation. In order to reach this level, you must have a profound understanding of the theory and abundant experience. Only then can you see far and predict the upcoming. Those who have reached only a low level of skill can merely defend themselves with an unsteady and unconfined mind all the time. In this case, they have already lost the battle. All of this depends on how well you have come to know the ways of creating and seizing opportunities.

Weighting Center

重
心

Every man has four limbs and a torso. The head is the leader, and the man's standing, bowing down, or looking upward, all have the head's postures. When the postures are firmed, then the weighting center (i.e., physical center) is established. When the weighting center is steady and firmed, it is said to have gained the advantageous situation and obtained the proper position. (If) the weighing center has lost its center, then there is a worry of falling. This means not gaining the advantageous situation and not obtaining the position. The fist techniques (i.e., martial arts), the foundation of the applications all depends on if the weighting center is steady and firmed. Furthermore, the weighting center can be distinguished as stationary or moving. The stationary one is, during the self-training fist techniques (i.e., martial techniques), to focus on every movement, every posture, all must be given attention all the time. (This also applies) to the turning, advancing or retreating.

凡人有四肢軀幹，頭為首，其站立俯仰，亦各有姿勢。姿勢立，則生重心。重心穩固，所謂得機得勢。重心失中，乃有顛倒之虞。即不得機，不得勢也。拳術，功用之基礎，則在重心之穩固與否。而重心又有固定與活動之分。固定者，是專主自己練習拳術之時，每一動作，一姿勢，均須時時注意之。或轉動，或進退皆然。

The mind is the leader of the entire body. It feels and controls the body's center and balance. When your mind and body can communicate with each other through sensing correctly, harmoniously, and comfortably, you can have a firmed center and the body will be in balance. When this happens, you have gained the advantageous situation and position for your action. However, if you cannot reach the above state of mind and body coordination, then you have lost your center and balance. Your root will be disrupted and the mind will be scattered and confused. In this case, you have lost the advantageous situation and position. The way of practicing this is first to start with stationary movements. Through every posture and movement, pay attention to the center and balance. After long practice, your mind's feeling will reach to a deep level. When this happens, the coordination of your mind and body will harmoniously and naturally follow. This stage is the regulating without regulating.

Weighting center, insubstantial and substantial originally belong to the same body (i.e., same subject). (However), the insubstantial and substantial can vary and without a regular pattern, the weighting center cannot (vary). (Even) though it is movable, because it is the master of the entire body, (it) cannot be moved without cautiousness which allows the opponent to know my insubstantial and substantial. It is just like in the battle. The heart (i.e., mind) is the order, the Qi is the message flag, and the waist is the banner. Taijiquan uses the (various) Jins as battle techniques, the insubstantial and substantial as battle tactics, Yi and Qi are the officers, Listening Jin is the spy, and weighting center is the commander.

重心與虛實本屬一體。虛實能變換無常，重心則不
然。雖能移動，因係全體之主宰，不能輕舉妄動，
使敵知吾虛實。又如作戰然。心為令，氣為旗，腰
為纛。太極拳以勁為戰術，虛實為戰略，意氣為指
揮，聽勁為間牒，重心為主帥。

In order to have insubstantial and substantial, you must first acquire firm balance and a weighted center. This implies not a heavy, dead center but one that is developed. Without the balance and center, your insubstantial and substantial will not grow from a firm root and your tactics will not be effective. This is because every movement of Taijiquan originates from the legs (i.e., root), is governed by the waist, and manifests through the fingers. Therefore, the firm root, which is generated from the balance and center, is the origin of the insubstantial and substantial action. That is why insubstantial and substantial can be varied, while the weight cannot change easily. If you change the root without caution, your enemy can feel and sense your intention and all of your tactics will be in vain.

It is just like in a battle. The Xin (i.e., emotional mind) initiates the idea of offense or defense which directs the Qi (message flag) to the physical body for Jin's manifestation. The waist controls the Jin and therefore is a banner. Different Jins offer different possibilities of skills. With the tactics of insubstantial and substantial variation and use of Yi (i.e., wisdom mind) to lead the Qi, listening Jin to gather intelligence, and also root as the command center, you can use your mind and entire body for battle effectively. Here, you must understand that Xin (i.e., emotional mind) initiates an action while Yi (i.e., wisdom mind) directs the action. They are equally important and must work harmoniously.

The practitioners (of Taijiquan) should ponder and comprehend these (matters) all the time. This is the entire great application of the Dao (of pushing hands). What is called the activities of the weighting center all depends on the comparison (i.e., situation) of the opponent and me (relatively). Though it is in the midst of combat, (you) must always keep (i.e., protect) your weighting center and attack the opponent's center. This is to protect the chief commander of the entire army and to fortify him against any disadvantage.

學者，應時時揣摸默識體會之。此為斯道全體大用
也。重心活動之謂，係在彼我相較之間，雖在決鬥
之中，必須時時維持自己之重心，而攻擊他人之重
心。即堅守全軍之司令，而不使主帥有所失利也。

This paragraph emphasizes the importance of protecting your center and balance, and destroying your opponent's center and balance. When you lose balance and root, you will not be able to execute your techniques and tactics effectively. This is also true for your opponent. Once your opponent has lost his balance and center, you will immediately grasp this opportunity to attack an exposed cavity.

雙重　Double Weighting

What is double weighting? It means there is no (discrimination of) insubstantial and substantial. The sickness (i.e., problem) of double weighting can be distinguished as single side or double sides and both hands and both legs. The classic says: "(When the opponent presses) sideward (or) downward, then follow. (When there is) double weighting (i.e., heaviness or mutual resistance), then (there is) stagnation." Also says: "Often, after several years of dedicated training, one still cannot apply this neutralization and is controlled by the opponent. (The reason for this is that the) fault of double heaviness is not understood." Therefore, the sickness (i.e., problem or mistake) of double weighting is the most difficult (problem) for someone to awaken to and comprehend. If not knowing the theory of the insubstantial and substantial, (it) is not easy to avoid (this problem). If (one) can solve this problem, then (he has) understood and comprehended the Listening Jin, touch and feel, insubstantial and substantial, question and answer, thoroughly.

雙重者，無虛實之謂也。雙重之病，有單方，與雙
方及兩手兩足之分。經云：〝偏沉則隨，雙重則滯
。〞又云：〝有數年純功而不能運用者，率為人制
，雙重之病未悟耳。〞故雙重之病，最難自悟自覺
。非知虛實之理，不易避免。能解此病，則聽勁、
感覺、虛實、問答皆能融會貫通焉！

Double weighting means when your opponent places a weight on you, you return with a weight. This will cause stagnation and mutual resistance. Double weighting can also be interpreted as you putting weight (i.e., force) on both of your hands at the same time without any insubstantial and substantial. Since the feet are the origins of the action, if the hands do not have the discrimination of insubstantial and substantial, it follows that your feet are also without insubstantial and substantial (i.e., double weighting).

Therefore, if you do not know what is insubstantial and substantial, most likely you will commit the problem of double weighting. When the opponent puts pressure on you, you must listen and follow (i.e., becoming insubstantial) without resistance (i.e., double weighting). In this case, you can avoid the double weighting of both sides. Furthermore, you must also avoid any double weighting generated from yourself. When both your hands apply pressure on the opponent at the same time, be sure the weight is not evenly distributed. This is double weighting. One can be less and the other one more. When this happens, you can change your insubstantial into substantial easily without being detected by your opponent. All of the success of avoiding double weighting depends on the development of your sensitive feeling (i.e., listening Jin) and how skillfully you can apply the tactics of insubstantial and substantial.

The reason that a bicycle can move and turn as is wished is all because of the scholar (i.e., principle) of mechanics. A person sits on the bicycle, the hands are handling (the bars) and the feet are stepping on the peddles, the eyes are looking, and the body is following. Its weighting center is on the waist which allows the body to look left and right and then use the hands to assist (the decision). Its turning wheel (i.e., the stepping wheel) is located at the center of the bicycle and the two feet are stepping on the peddles, one steps and one lifts, then the wheel turns the chain (to move) the wheels and move forward. If both feet step with effort at the same time, then the bicycle will stop going forward. This is because of the problem of double weighting.

腳踏車之所以能行動灣轉自如者，均力學也。人坐
於車上，手拂之，足踏之，目視之，身隨之，其重
心在腰，而司顧盼，以手輔助之。其輪盤置於車之
中心，兩足踏於腳蹬之上，一踏一提，則輪齒絞鍊
而帶動前進矣。若兩足同時用力踏之，則車即停止
前進，此蓋雙重之病耳。

The way to ride a bicycle is similar to the theory of self double weighting. You must balance yourself in the seat (center) and maintain equilibrium, applying energy to both sides evenly without discrimination of insubstantial and substantial.

It is the same in pushing hands. (If) the opponent uses force to push me and I also use force to resist, then both are mutually resist. This is called stagnation. This is the double weighting of both sides. If I or the opponent (know how to) follow the coming force, do not resist with force, and retreat by following the opponent's force and lead it farther, in addition, with the skills of no losing and resisting, then there must be one side's force lost into emptiness. This is accomplished because of (the trick) of following (the opponent's pressure) and leading it sideward (or) downward.

夫推手亦然。對方用力推我，吾若仍以力相抵抗之
，因而相持，則謂之滯。此即雙方之雙重也。若我
或彼，各順其勢，不以力抵抗，而順對方來力之方
向撤回，引之前進。然須不丟不頂，則必有一方之
力落空。此即偏沉所致。

In pushing hands with an opponent, if you resist against an incoming force, it is double weighting on both sides. When this happens, the Qi and the force become stagnant. The key to handling the incoming force is to lead it sideward and downward. When this happens, you have led his force into emptiness.

(For the case), I wish to attack the opponent's side and make him fall. If I use both hands to push (the opponent) directly and the opponent's power is strong, (I) would not be able to defeat his force. (In this case, I) must use the method of insubstantial and substantial. Use both of my hands to touch his shoulders, my left hand rolling downward his right shoulder while my right hand attacks (i.e., pushes) his left shoulder. At this time, my hands are in the posture of mutual support and aim to the same direction to form the Jin into a circle. In this case, the opponent('s body) will slant and fall. This is because the opponent cannot handle the situations both on the top and the bottom simultaneously and has lost his advantageous position. This is also caused due to my Jin's emitting sideward and downward. The practitioners (once) comprehend one will know ten. (This is) from mastering (the skill of insubstantial and substantial) and gradually comprehending the Understanding Jin.

如我擬攻對方之側面，使其倒地。若以兩手直接推之，而對方力氣強大，不可挫其鋒，須以虛實之法，雙手撫其肩，我左手由彼之右肩下擺，同時我右手擊其左肩，此時我兩手作交叉之勢，同主一方，而發勁成一圓形，則彼可側斜而倒，因彼同時不能上下相顧，而失利也。此即吾發勁偏沉所致也。學者悟一而知十。所謂由著熟，而漸悟懂勁也。

For example, if you wish to make someone fall, you cannot push both of your hands directly toward him. This is because using both of your hands like this is double weighting, and your opponent has great potential to generate power to resist you. This is a double weighting of yourself and also with your opponent. The best way to make your opponent lose his balance is first to contact both his shoulders with both of your hands. One hand is pulling one side down while the other is pushing the other side up. In this case, you have generated an insubstantial and substantial leverage to make him fall. If you can comprehend this theory, you can apply it to other situations. The more you practice, the better you can do. This is the way of Understanding Jin.

Giving Up Self and Following Opponent

捨己從人

To give up myself and follow the opponent is to abandon my idea and follow the opponent's movements. This is the most difficult thing (i.e., training) in Taijiquan. Because when two persons are exchanging hands (i.e., combatting), the conception of wining and losing is serious. (In this case) the opponent and I will not endure each other, not even mentioning that when mutually (we) are attacking each other or mutually stalemating with each other and (you) are asked to give up your right (of trying to win in a resisting competition). What is called to give up yourself and follow the opponent is not only explained from the words. In our Dao (i.e., the Dao of Taijiquan), its hidden meaning is extremely profound. (In order to understand them and apply them in action,) the practitioner must put a Gongfu in the four words: solely focus in cultivating the human nature.

捨己從人，是捨棄自己的主張，而依從他人動作。
在太極拳中，為最難能之事。因兩人在交手之時，
勝負之觀念重，彼我決不相容，何況互相攻擊，或
在相持之中，而棄其權利。所謂捨己從人，不僅作
字面解釋而矣。在吾道中，其寓意至深。學者當於
惟務養性，四字下功夫。

The most difficult training in Taijiquan pushing hands is to follow and adhere with the opponent's movement. Do not lose contact and do not resist. This is trained quite a lot, but in reality, it is still very difficult. This is because when both you and your opponent are resisting each other, the ego of winning is strong. Only if you can give up this ego can you listen and follow the opponent's intention. When this happens, you can lead your opponent's energy into emptiness and make his intention in vain. The first crucial key to training this is to cultivate your human nature. Human nature here means the ego, impatience, and emotional intention. Only through disciplined cultivation and a release of such mental, emotional and spiritual tension can you learn the secret of influencing your opponent's intention. Sun Tzu (子) says that the highest form of strategy is to strike the opponent's will. This is an aspect of such high strategy.

The classics say: "(Taiji is) generated from Wuji, and is a pivotal function of movement and stillness. It is the mother of Yin and Yang." (The action of) movement and calmness is human nature, (the concept of) Yin and Yang is the theory. Therefore, human nature and the theory are the original source of the Dao. The saying of cultivating human nature is where the practitioner should place the effort at all times. Contemplate and ponder deeply in the heart, the heart (i.e., mind) grasps the meaning and the spirit meets (i.e., concentrates), after a long time, (one) will comprehend the meaning suddenly. It also says: "From mastering (the techniques of adhering and following), then you can gradually grasp what "Understanding Jin (Dong Jin)" means. From "Understanding Jin," you gradually approach enlightenment (intuitive understanding) of your opponent's intention." This is the theory of repeated cycling and returning (all the training) to its origin. This is what is called "beyond appearance and having gained the position in the ring." When training Gongfu to the refined and precise (level), (then you) can create the opportunity without worry about unable to obtain the advantageous position, are capable of bending and extending as wish everywhere. Then there is no disadvantage wherever you go. In this case, (you) can give up yourself and follow the opponent.

經云：〝無極而生，動靜之機，陰陽之母也。〞動
靜為性，陰陽為理。故性理為道之本源。養性之說
，是學者應時時致力修養，潛心揣摩，心領神會，
久之自能豁然貫通矣。又云：〝由著熟而漸悟懂勁
，懂勁後而階及神明。〞此乃循環之理，歸宗之意
。蓋所謂超以象外，得其寰中。功夫練到精微，能
造機造勢，不愁無得機得勢處。能處處隨曲就伸，
則無往不利。如此乃能捨己從人。

In Wang, Zong-Yue's *Taijiquan Classic*, he said: "What is Taiji?
It is generated from Wuji, and is a pivotal function of movement and
stillness. It is the mother of Yin and Yang. When it moves, it divides.
At rest it reunites." From this, you can see that Taiji is not Wuji (i.e.,
no extremity), nor is it Yin and Yang, but is between the Wuji and the
Yin-Yang division. That means Taiji is actually the force or the motivation which makes the Wuji derive into Yin-Yang and vice versa.

For example, when you practice Taijiquan, the initial, still and
stationary posture is the Wuji state. Once you start to move, Yin and
Yang are derived from Wuji and discriminated. In this case, what
makes you move from Wuji to Yin-Yang is called Taiji. Naturally,
you can perceive that it is the mind which makes you move.
Therefore, when the Taiji concept is applied to human action, the
mind is the motivator or the origin of all action. That means the Taiji
is our mind.

When the mind is manifested into action, the decision of movement or calmness is from inside. The manner of its manifestation
into Yin or Yang external form follows this theory. Therefore, human
thinking and its creation of Yin and Yang manifestations is the gate-
way of the Dao. From this, you can see that the deeper and more
profound levels that your mind can reach, the more refined, elegant
and effective actions can be manifested. If you cannot comprehend
this theory, it does not matter how hard you practice, the effort will
be in vain. This is simply because the theory is the foundation of the
action, and the theory originates from the mind.

After the theory (i.e., understanding of mind) has been manifested into external Yin-Yang action, you must practice all the time until
you have mastered the skills. The more you ponder, the more you
practice, and the more you will understand. This is the way of com-

prehending the key to "Understanding Jin." Understanding Jin follows after "Listening Jin" (i.e., feeling). The more sensitively you can feel the opponent, the more you can understand his intention. After you have practiced for a long time, you will reach the stage where, if your opponent moves just slightly, you already know his intention. If you can reach a deeper level of listening and understanding Jin, then even before your opponent's intention is manifested externally, you can sense it. In this case, you have reached the enlightened stage of practice.

Once you have reached this stage, you can create opportunities without worrying about having to gain an advantageous position. When this happens, you can move and act as you wish. This means you can give yourself up and follow the opponent anywhere and anytime.

————————————

Drumming and Vibrating

鼓盪

The Qi is sunken, the waist is loose, the abdomen is clear, the chest is contained, the back is arced, the shoulder is sunken, the elbow is dropped. Every section is comfortable and extensive (i.e., loose and relaxed). Moving, calmness, insubstantial, substantial, exhaling, inhaling, opening, closing, hardening, softening, slow, fast, all of these mixed Jins are drumming and vibrating. It is varied (i.e., derived) from the threading (i.e., connection) of the heart (i.e., mind) and Qi. It is like the huge wind and scary wave, hard to predict the wind and the cloud (i.e., weather). Taiji pushing hands, the last stage of Gongfu is called "Random Picking up Flowers," also named "Pick up the Wave Flower," all depends on the Jin of drumming and vibration. To agitate the opponent and make him stay in the position as a boat encountering the wind in the ocean, entering and exiting within the waves, dizzy and no mastering, slant and crumble, losing the self weighting center, hard to figure out (the situation), this is the function (i.e., consequence) of drumming and vibration.

氣沉、腰鬆、腹淨、含胸、拔背、沉肩、垂肘。節節舒展。動之，靜之、虛之、實之、呼之、吸之、開之、合之、剛之、柔之、緩之、急之。此種混合之勁，乃是鼓盪也。由心氣貫串，陰陽變化而來。如颶風駭浪，風雲莫測者也。太極推手，最後工夫有爛採花者，又名「採浪花」，全以鼓盪之勁，鼓動對方，使之如海船遇風，出入波濤之中，眩暈無主，頃斜顛簸，自身重心，難以捉摸。即鼓盪之作用也。

In order to make your Qi full like a drum that can generate a strong noise through great vibration, you must first have a calm and steady mind. When this mind leads the Qi to sink in the Lower Dan Tian, you will be rooted and balanced. Once you have full Qi in the Lower Dan Tian and firm root and balance, then you can regulate your body as such: the waist is loose, the abdomen is clear, the chest is contained, the back is arced, the shoulders are sunk, the elbows are dropped. Every section is loose, relaxed, and comfortable. In addition, you can regulate your breathing and mind to set up Yin and Yang strategies such as: moving, calmness, insubstantial, substantial, exhaling, inhaling, opening, closing, hardening, softening, slow, fast etc. When you apply the internal concentrated mind and abundant Qi to conditioned external action, the Jins manifested and the strategies executed will be effective and powerful. This is because all of the actions originate from the mind and the Qi, and apply to Yin and Yang strategies.

When your opponent encounters you, he will soon realize that he does not have any choice in any action. His mind is confused and scattered and his actions are not controllable. He feels like he is lost in the huge storm and cannot firm his root and balance. If you can reach this stage of Gongfu, it is called "Random Picking up Flowers," or "Pick up the Wave Flower."

Foundation

基礎

Taijiquan uses the fist frames (i.e., postures) as the body (i.e., major training subject) and the pushing hands as the applications. At the beginning, in learning (to) entwine the frame (i.e., basic stances and movements), the foundation is the most important. The posture must be accurate, centered, upright, peaceful, and comfortable. The movements must be slow but light, agile, round and alive. This is the path of entering the door (i.e., learning). The learner should advance following the order so (he/she) will not waste the Gongfu (i.e., energy and time) but able to gain the path short-cut.

太極拳以拳架為體，以推手為用。在初學盤架時，基礎最關重要。其姿勢務求正確，而中正安舒。其動作必須緩和，而輕靈圓活。此係入門之徑。學者循序而進，不致妄費功夫，而得其捷徑也。

The main training of Taijiquan is the thirty-seven postures. From these postures, the techniques are derived. Once you understand and master the techniques, you apply them into pushing hands. From pushing hands practice, you will gradually know how to apply the techniques to an opponent.

However, when you just start to learn Taijiquan, you must focus on the fundamental stances and basic movements. Here, you should understand "Pan Jia" (盤架) means "entwine the frame" in Chinese. It is common terminology in Chinese martial arts. At the beginning of your practice, you learn how to squat down to firm your root (i.e., fundamental stances) and to practice the basic physical movements to build up a foundation. All of these trainings are called "Pan Jia." The fundamental stances are the foundation of all Taijiquan movements. With the solid foundation of the fundamental stances, you will have a firm root, center, and balance. In order to reach these goals, your body must be upright and comfortable. The movements should be slow, which allows you to think and understand. However, the most important element of all is allowing yourself to feel the postures. Once you can feel the movements, you can make them light, agile, and round. The best way of approaching these requirements is learning, understanding, practicing, and feeling, step by step. This is the short-cut of reaching the final goal. If you do not follow this path, you will build up many bad habits and it will take you a longer time, with more mistaken turns that will require correction over time.

What is the center? (First,) the Xin (i.e., emotional mind) and the Qi must be centered and harmonious, the spirit is clear and the Qi is sunken. The root is in the feet, that is the key point of standing. The weight center is linked (i.e., related) to the waist and spine. This is what is said, the origin of the life-Yi (i.e., crucial key to life) is on the waist. The spirit should be contained and condensed internally without manifesting externally. Then (you) can be centered, steady, sunken, and calm. What is upright? The postures are accurate and upright. (That means) every posture must be correct and proper, taboo the leaning and slant. However, (there are) many kinds of postures and are all different, either facing upward, bowing down, extending, or bending, not all centered and upright. Therefore, their Jin's manifestation and the intention of the mind all demand for the weight center. This is because the weight center is the main hinge of the entire body. When the weight center is established, then opening and closing can be agile and alive as wish. If the weight center is not established, the opening and closing will lose its key point. It is like the axle is the major hinge of the wheels. If this axle is out of alignment and is not located at the weight center area, then when the wheels are turning, the advancing and backward will lose their effectiveness. Therefore, the postures of the fist frame (i.e., structure) must be accurate, consequently, the weight center will be balanced and steady. Otherwise, the weight center will be shifted and your insubstantial and substantial will be seen clearly.

中者，心氣中和，神清氣沉。其根在腳，即是立點。重心繫於腰脊。所謂命意源頭在腰隙，精神含斂於內，不表於外。乃能中定沉靜矣。正者，姿勢端正。每一姿勢，務宜端正，而忌偏斜。然各種姿勢，各不相同。或仰、或俯、或伸、或屈、非盡中正。是以其發勁，及其用意之方向，而求其重心。蓋重心為全體樞紐。重心立，則開合靈活自如。重心不立，則開合失其關鍵。如車軸為車輪之樞紐。若使車軸，置於偏斜，而不適於車身之重心處，則車輪轉動，進退失其效用矣。故拳架之姿勢，務求正確，則重心平穩。要不自牽扯其重心，而辨別虛實也。

Your ability to keep your physical center is initially determined by your ability to keep your mental center. In order to keep your mental center, first you must build up a deep feeling to feel it. When the feeling is deep and profound, the mental center will be refined to a deep stage. When this happens, the mental center and the physical center can coordinate with each other and finally reach the goal of balancing both mentally and physically. From this, you can see that sensitive feeling is the key to reaching the centered state. In order to achieve a deep feeling, you must first have a calm mind and harmonious Qi circulation. With the calm mind and harmonious Qi circulation, your feeling will be accurate and refined. In this case you will have a firm balance and center.

After you have a firm center and balance, you should build up a firm root. Again, a firm root is built based on how deeply your feeling can reach. You must train the sensitive feeling of your feet to find the way of connecting to the ground and creating a root. Once you have a good centered, balanced, and rooted mental and physical body, then you have built up a firm foundation for pushing hands.

However, in action it is not enough that you just can keep your center and firm your root. You must know how to find the center where the Jins are controlled. If you cannot comprehend this action center, even if you have a great mental and physical center, once in motion you will immediately lose balance. Therefore, when the center and root are mentioned, this passage is not just talking about a stationary center and root. It is talking about the center and the root of the action. That means the center and root for the Jins' manifestation.

It is said in *Taiji Classic* that the Jins originate from the feet, are directed by the waist and are finally manifested in the fingers. This means that in order to have powerful and effective Jin manifestation, you must have a firm root from the feet, and also a well controlled waist which can direct the Jin as you wish. From there, you can see that the center of the Jin's manifestation is in the waist. It is just like a car; the steering wheel that controls and directs the entire car's movement is the waist in Taijiquan. The engine is the power source and is in the feet, and the wheels are the fingers in Taijiquan.

The most important key to successful Jin manifestation is the spirit. When the spirit is high, the Qi is strong and the mind is concentrated. In this case, the Jin manifested will be powerful. However, when the spirit is high, it does not mean you are excited. When the spirit is excited, the mind cannot concentrate, and the Jin cannot be focused. Therefore, although the spirit is high, still it must be condensed (i.e., restrained) internally. When this happens, you are really centered both physically and mentally. This will provide you with an advantage for strategic insubstantial and substantial actions.

What is the peace? Means peaceful and easy. Be sure not coercive and forceful. (When all postures) are originated from the natural way, then (they) can be peaceful and comfortable. Therefore, it will not have the problem of Qi's stagnation and can circulate the Qi around the entire body. This is because the postures are peaceful and steady, the movements are uniform, the breathing is peaceful and harmonious, and the spirit and Qi are calm and quiet.

安者，安然之意。切忌牽強。由自然之中，得其安
適，乃無氣滯之弊，而能氣遍身軀矣。此由於姿勢
安穩，動作均勻，呼吸平和，神氣鎮靜所致。

The peace means the mind is calm, harmonious, and comfortable. When this mind is manifested externally, your physical body
will be relaxed, the breathing will be peaceful and harmonious, and
consequently, the movements will be natural. When this happens,
the best condition for the Qi's circulation is provided. Once your Qi
can circulate to the entire body, your feeling will be sensitive and
accurate. This is because the feeling of the body and the mind are
connected through the nervous system, and the vitality and the function of the nervous system depends on the Qi supply (i.e., bioelectric-
ity supply). Feeling is a language between our mind and body.

---

*What is the comfort? (It) means comfortable and exten-
sive. Therefore, it is said, first ask for the opening and
extending and then ask for the tightening and closing.
At the beginning of learning entwine the frame (i.e.,
basic movements), the postures and the movements
first aiming for opening and extensive and making all
the joints in the entire body comfortable and extended.
However, it does not mean to extend the tendons and
bones (i.e., joints) by Li (i.e., muscular force) on purpose. (They should) be fluidly and naturally extended
gradually. After a long time (of practice), (the postures)
will be relaxed, alive, and steady naturally.*

舒者，舒展之謂。故云先求開展，後求緊湊。初學
盤架時，姿勢動作，務求開展。使全體關節，節節
舒展之。然非故意用力伸張筋骨。於自然之中，徐
徐鬆展。久之自然鬆活沉著矣。

When your joints can be extended and relaxed, you will feel comfortable. When the joints are tightened, they will be locked. Consequently, the Qi will be stagnant. Therefore, it is said: "Taijiquan starts with large and low postures and reaches higher with small and high postures." This is because if you would like to feel deeply into the joints, you must first learn how to extend the joints. Only if you can extend them comfortably can you then relax them to a profound stage. However, to make all of this happen, do not rely on muscular force. It is accomplished from breathing, the mind's feeling and the relaxation of the joints.

What is the lightness? (It) means light and insubstantial. However, be sure not coercive and forceful, not to be drift and float. When practice the entwine frame (i.e., basic movements), the movements must be light and agile, to and fro can then be (executed) as wished. After a long time, the Jin of looseness and aliveness will be automatically generated and advanced into the birth of the Jins of sticking (i.e., connecting) and adhering. Therefore, the word of lightness is the beginning of practicing Taijiquan and the path of entering the door.

輕者，輕虛之意。然忌漂浮。在盤架時，動作要輕
靈而和緩，往復乃能自如。久之自生鬆活之勁，進
而生粘黏之勁。故輕字是練太極拳下手之處，入門
之途徑。

The lightness here does not mean the body is light. What it says is the contact between you and your opponent should be light instead of heavy. When it is heavy, it will be forceful and therefore generating double weighting (i.e., mutual resistance) easily. Not only that, when it is heavy, the feeling will be shallow and this will prevent you from communicating (i.e., listening Jin) with your opponent clearly.

However, the contact between you and your opponent should not be too light and floating. When this happens, you can easily lose contact with the opponent. After you have trained for a long time, you will be skillful enough to initiate a light touch without losing your opponent. This is what is called: "Do not lose and resist." This is the Jin of sticking (i.e., attachment) and adherence. From this, you can see that learning to touch lightly without losing and resisting is the first step in learning Taiji pushing hands.

What is the agility? (It) means agile and sensitive (in feeling). From light and insubstantial to loosing and sunken, from loosing and sentineling to sticking (i.e., attaching) and adhering. (If you) can stick and adhere, then can connect (i.e., keep in touch) and follow. (If you) can connect and follow, then (you) can be agile and sensitive. (In this case), then (you) can comprehend (the skills of) no losing and no resisting.

靈者，靈敏之謂。由輕虛而鬆沉，由鬆沉而粘黏。
能粘黏，即能連隨。能連隨，而後方能靈敏，則可
悟及不丟不頂矣。

Agility means the capability of corresponding with the opponent's action smoothly, accurately, and with agility. However, in order to reach this goal, you must first learn to be light and insubstantial. Insubstantial here implies that you are ready for quick response. If you are in a substantial situation, then your mind has already been manifested and you are in an offensive state. When you initiate a light attachment with your opponent, you must be open and ready for any action. Therefore, your mind must be insubstantial.

In order to be agile, first you must be able to attach to the opponent lightly and fluidly, then you learn to be loose and sunken. This means to attach firmly. Only then will you be able to connect and adhere with the opponent. After you have learned the skills of connecting, you will be able to follow. Once you have mastered the skill of following, you will be able to react with fluid agility. When this time comes, will you really comprehend what is the meaning of not losing and not resisting.

What is the roundness? (It) means round and full. In every posture and every movement, (you) must ask for round and full (i.e., complete and perfect) and no defect, then (you) can be integrated with a sole Qi and avoid the problem of deficiency and sufficiency and continuity and break. (When you) apply different Jins in the pushing hands, if it is not round, then not agile. (If it) can be round, the it can be alive. (If) everywhere can be alive, then there is no place with disadvantages.

圓者，圓滿之謂。每一姿勢一動作，務求圓滿，而無缺陷，則能完整一氣。而免凸凹斷續之病。推手運用各勁，非圓不靈。能圓則活。處處能活，則無往不利。

Round means each movement should be continuous and perfect. Without continuing and then breaking and vice visa. If you can perform every movement smoothly and continuously, then you have the feeling of completeness. Once you have this feeling, your breathing will be smooth and natural. When this happens, the Qi can be led by the mind strongly and perfectly. Taijiquan was created based on the principle of neutralization. When you move with roundness, it is easier to be continuous. This means it is easier for your neutralization. Most neutralizing is accomplished from yielding and leading through round movements. If you can comprehend this concept, then your actions will be alive without disadvantages.

What is the aliveness? (It) means agile and alive. That means there is no clumsy, heavy, delay, and stagnant. After you have threaded through (i.e., comprehend thoroughly) all of the above described paragraphs, then there is nothing without freedom in extending, bending, opening, and closing, advancing, retreating, bowing, and facing upward. That is what is meant, (if you) can breathe, then (you) can be agile and alive.

活者，靈活之謂。無笨重遲滯之意。上述各節，貫
通後，則伸屈開合，進退俯仰，無不自由。所謂能
呼吸，而後能靈活也。

As explained above, the final goal of practicing your movement in action is looking for the aliveness and agility of the skills and techniques. This means the techniques can be executed naturally and smoothly as you wish. You must comprehend all of what has been described above. When this happens, every movement and action can be performed without tension. Once you can execute the techniques fluidly, without tension and stagnation, your breathing can be smooth and natural. Only then can you be really agile and alive.

授
受

Teaching and Learning

All human personalities are different from each other. Generally speaking, they can be divided into two kinds: call them hard and soft. The personality of hardness is urgent and aggressive. With high (morality), it means strong, and with low (morality), it becomes violent. Those strong like to contend (i.e., compete or argue), therefore, when they learn the fist like to focus on the hardness. It is because their personality likes to compete with strength and struggling for winning, not willing to be under other people. Those soft (persons), the personality is peaceful and smooth (i.e., harmonious). With high morality, their heart (i.e., mind) and Qi harmonious and deeply respect others. Therefore, when they learn the fist, they like to be soft. This is because their personalities like peace and have an open-minded nature. Those violent, the personality is impatient and rude. Therefore, when they learn the fist, like to focus on the fierce and lack of interest in pursuing refined and deeper level. Those soft and with low (morality), the personality is too soft and weak, the will is not strong, lack of the aggressive mind. Therefore, when learning the fist, do not search for the deep and profound meaning.

夫人之性情，各有不同，大抵可分為兩種。曰剛、
與柔是也。剛性急而烈，上者為強，下者為暴。強
者喜爭，故其學拳時多務於剛，以其性喜爭強鬥勝
，不屈人下也。柔者性和而順，上者心氣中和而篤
敬。故其學拳時，多務於柔。以其性喜和平多涵養
也。暴者，性燥而魯莽。故其學拳時，專務於猛，
而無精細之趣。柔之下者，性柔而弱，意志不強，
少進取心，故學拳時不求甚解。

When you teach Taijiquan, first analyze your student. What is the motivation for his learning? What kind of personality does he have? Is he patient? Has he strong will and perseverance? Will you waste your time with this student? In China, it is said: "A master will spend three years to test a student." From testing, you can see if a student is worthy to be taught. If not, you simply waste your time and energy. The student you are looking for is a student who has a strong will, is patient, perseveres, and can be strong both mentally and physically and also calm when it is necessary. He is humble to learn, and enjoys pondering deeply and challenging himself.

It is the same if you are a student. First, you must analyze yourself. Is your personality suitable for what you want to learn? Very often, what you want to learn is not what you are capable of learning. Once the honeymoon period is over, you will lose your interest and try something else. If you are impatient like that and lack a strong commitment, then you will simply waste your time and energy. Naturally, you will not be taken seriously by your teacher.

However, a martial artist should be precious in the hard will (i.e., strong will) and the personality should be soft. (He should also) have wisdom, kindness, and bravery, then the hard and the soft can be supporting each other mutually. In this case, (he) can improve his morality and advance (his) study. The above description about personality is related to the human nature of the learner, (you) should be aware of it. Due to the different personalities of the learners, the results they have achieved are also different. (I) observe these when (I) have leisure time. Those who learn Taijiquan, though originated from the same teacher, their postures of the fist (i.e., Taijiquan) and the explanation of the theory are all different. Therefore, it has passed down many doubts and misunderstandings. All of these are created because the teacher who taught the students adapted to the student's personality. This is what is meant "a slight error can cause a thousand-mile divergence." Therefore, (I) mentioned here specially, so as to explain the doubts of the people, and to be a reference.

然武人貴志剛而性柔，有智、有仁、有勇，方為剛
柔相濟。如此乃能進德修業矣。上述性別，關乎學
者之本性，應注意之。學者以性情之不同，而所得
結果亦異。間嘗竊觀，學太極拳者，雖同一師承，
而其拳之姿勢，與理論之解釋各異，因而遺下多少
竇疑及誤會。凡此蓋亦教授者因其人之性情而授受
耳。所謂差之毫釐，謬以千里。故特表而出之，以
解釋群疑，而資參考焉。

Therefore, as a martial artist, you should understand yourself and improve both your personality and morality. Dare to accept the challenge and dare to admit the mistakes you have committed. Be humble, kind and willing to learn, and ponder to increase your wisdom. In this case, you will acquire both the Yin and Yang sides of personality. You will soon be a successfully proficient Taijiquan practitioner.

Appendix A: The Thesis of Taijiquan—Questions and Answers by Xiang, Kai-Ran[*]

About Xiang, Kai-Ran. Xiang, Kai-Ran (1889-1957 A.D.), also named Xiang, Kui (向逵), nickname Bu Xiao Sheng (不肖生); Ancestors were living at Ping Jiang, Hunan Province (湖南・平江). However, he was born at Xiang Tan (湘潭). He liked Wushu since he was young and was also interested in scholarship. First, he learned Wu family style (巫家拳) Wushu. In 1905 he went to Japan to study politics and law. While he was in Japan, he practiced Wushu with a Chinese student Wang, Zhi-Qun (王志群). In 1911, he returned to China and was employed as a military judge in Chang Sa (長沙). In 1913, he again went to Japan to study in the Japanese Central University in Tokyo (日本東京中央大學). After he returned from Japan in 1917, he founded "The Chinese Fist Techniques Research Institute" (中華拳術研究會). He has written many books and novels such as: *Fist Techniques* (拳術), *The Passage of Fist Techniques* (拳術傳薪錄), *The Seeing and Hearing of Fist Techniques* (拳術見聞), etc.

A guest who has doubts about Taijiquan said: "The applications of the fist (i.e., martial arts) are to combat with the opponent. All men have the same four limbs and hundred skeletons. If wish to win (the battle), why do we give up the speed and the strength? Therefore, there is a saying in the fist society (i.e., martial society) that (if) one is fast, cannot be defeated, and (if) one is hard (i.e., strong) can not be worsted. However, today's Taijiquan practitioners say, not to use the force as the body (i.e., main emphasis) and use the slow as the applications. Don't these sayings conflict with the theory of fist theory?"

[*]*Chinese Wushu Great Dictionary* (〔中一國武術大辭典〕，人民體育出版社。), 1990.

太極拳論—問答　向愷然

69

客有致疑於太極拳者曰：〝拳之為用，主搏人，四
肢百骸，人同所具，欲操勝算，捨快與力奚由。故
拳家有一快不破，一硬不破之言。乃今言之太極拳
者，則曰：〝以不用力為體，以慢為用〞，得毋與
拳之原理相悖謬乎？〞

*I said: "True. As to the applications of the fist, there is
no reason to give up the strength and the speed. Aren't
you going to say that those whose fists are fast and powerful are better than Taijiquan?"*

余曰：〝誠然，拳之為用，捨力與快無由。客將謂
拳之快而多力者，有逾於太極拳者乎？〞

*The guest said: "I have practiced Taijiquan for three
years. The (Taijiquan) ancestors always told us: 'once
move, the entire body must be light and agile. Using the
Jin like drawing silk, should not be broken and then continue, etc. Don't all of these sayings mean (Taijiquan)
should be (practiced) slow and not using strength? I
ponder this theory day and night, without gap (i.e.,
break) winter and summer. However, I used to compete
(i.e., sparring) with a martial artist in (my) village who
had just learned other fist (i.e., martial art) only a few
months. I was always defeated and did not know how to
handle the situation. Therefore, in the past I doubted
that it (i.e., Taijiquan) was the skill which could be used
for fighting. More and more, I believe it is true. Now,
you told me those (martial artists) whose fists are faster
and more powerful cannot compete (with Taijiquan
martial artist), I would like to hear the reasons."*

客曰：「吾習太極拳三年於茲矣。先哲嘗詔吾曰：
『一舉動週身俱要輕靈，用勁如抽絲，不可斷續。』
是云云者，非慢而不用力之謂乎？吾寢饋其中，
無間寒燠。然嘗與里中之習他拳才數月者角，輒敗
退不知所以支吾之道，曩固疑其非搏人之術。茲益
信其然矣。今吾子顧曰：『拳之快而多力者，無逾
比。』願聞其說。」

I said: "Strange! What you said about fast and hard,
aren't they the arms' bending and extending, the feet's
fast forward and backward, the coarse muscles and skin,
the tendons' and bones' strength and solidity as the hardness? These are the natural talents of human. They are
not related to the cultivation of the arts. Furthermore,
the bending and extending, advancing and retreating,
their applications are very simple. Though they are fast,
they must have some gaps which allow the opponent to
take the opportunity. The applications of Taijiquan,
though also not separate from bending, extending,
advancing, and retreating, however, are searching for
the straight among the bending. Its appearance is like
roundness, only it is round, then its applications will
not be restricted in a single way.

余曰：「異哉！子之所謂快與硬也，豈不以手之屈
伸，足之進退為快，肌膚之粗糙，筋骨之堅實為硬
乎？是屬於人類自然之本能，無關藝術之修養者也
。且屈伸進退，為用甚簡。雖至迅，必有間，人得
而乘焉。太極拳之為用，雖亦不離乎屈伸進退，然
曲中求直，其象如圜。唯其圜也，為用不拘一方。

It is just like the applications of a spear. Everyone
knows (its applications) are on the tip. Everyone also
knows the applications of a saber are on the sharp blade

as well. Isn't it as simple as such! However, the applications of the roundness, it can be there or not there (i.e., substantial or insubstantial). This is because its applications can be existing everywhere. Therefore, every movement of the body must be light and agile. There is almost no sickness (i.e., no difficulty) as other fists (i.e., martial styles) those who learn the fist but hard to apply the fist and those who learn the hips and hard to apply the feet. Comparing with other fists, its speed and swiftness are hard to be counted by number. The fist classic says: "Each place has each place's insubstantial and substantial. Everywhere all relies on these insubstantial and substantial." It also says: "Once moves, no place without moving, once calm, no place without calm." Therefore, it is understood that the applications of every movement are numerous and profound.

猶之槍之為用，人知其在穎也。刀之為用，人知其在鋒也。非甚簡矣乎！若夫圓之為用，則無在無不在也。唯其用之無不在也。故一舉動週身俱要輕靈。庶幾無習於拳者，難於掌。習於臀者，難於足之病。其迅捷視他拳不可以數字計。拳經載，一處有一處虛實，處處總此一虛實。又謂，一動無有不動，一靜無有不靜。是可知其一舉動為用之繁賾矣。

Other fists, seldom or do not use the broken Jins. When broken and then continue, the gap (i.e., opportunity) will be given to the opponent. Taijiquan eliminates the trace of the breaking and continuing. When applied, it can be broken any time as wished, after broken can be connected again. Wang, Zong-Yue said: 'Attaching is yielding and yielding is attaching. The opponent does not know me but I know the opponent.' This is what it means. After practice for a long time then can reach the refined stage. Try to think, when there is a movement that is applied to the entire body, then everywhere must examine the place (i.e., situation) of insubstantial and substantial carefully. Then when it is manifested externally, how can it not be slow."

他拳鮮不用斷勁者。斷而復續，授隙於人。太極拳泯斷續之跡，用之隨在可斷，斷而復連。王宗岳謂：〝粘即是走，走即是粘，人不知我，我獨知人。〞正是於此等處。用力久而後能臻於縝密。試思一舉動之為用遍週身，處處皆當詳審其虛實所在，則其形於外者，安得不慢乎！〞

The guest said: "Now, I have heard the Dao (i.e., theory) of the slow. May I also hear the saying of using no force against multiple force (i.e., strong force)?"

客曰：〝慢之道，得聞命矣。其以無力為多力之說，可得聞乎？〞

I said: "The fist techniques do not value (i.e., pay attention) in Li (i.e., muscular force), but value in Jin. This is not only applied in Taijiquan. (In fact,) all of the fist techniques are like this. This is because a person (i.e., martial artist) does not worry about without (i.e., lacking of) Li but worries about his Li not being concentrated. Therefore, even those people without Li, an arm's weight is 10 kilograms. (If he) can bend and extend for exercises, then each of his arm has the Li of 10 kilograms. A body's weight is several 10 kilograms, however, (I) have never heard (one) who is unable to lift his foot by himself. Then, his feet has the Li of several 10 kilograms. These are all acquired by those weakest persons in the heaven and earth (i.e., world). But these are the Li and not Jin. (These) cannot concentrate to a single point and be transmitted into the opponent's body. Therefore, they are not valuable. Those practicing fists should be able to transform the Li into Jin.

余曰：〝拳術不貴力，而貴勁。不僅太極拳也。一
切拳術，則皆然矣。夫人不患無力，特患其力之不
能集中耳。力為人所恆有。世故無力之人，一臂之
重十斤。能屈伸運動，則一臂具十斤之力矣。一身
之重數十斤，未聞其足不能自舉，則足具數十斤之
力矣。此為天下至弱者之所同具，但以其為力而非
勁也。不能集中一點，以傳達於敵人之身，故不足
貴。習拳者，在使力化為勁。

If (you) can gather 10 kilograms of Jin into the hands and attack the opponent, the opponent must be injured. Several 10 kilograms are concentrated at the foot and strike the opponent, the opponent must be dead. In this case, why worry about not enough Li for use. The appearance of other fists, the palms are palms, the elbows are elbows, it is known easily and obviously. However, the practitioners have practiced for a long time and become habit. Most of them still have the coarse and stiffness and cannot concentrate their Jin and reach the opponent. The sickness (i.e., problem) of this is knowing Li as the Li and not knowing the no Li as the Li. Grabbing the fist (so powerful) and showing the claws, biting the teeth (so strong) as if penetrating to the gums, still look it as a martial strength and do not know the Li has collapsed into the shoulders and back and become an opportunity for the opponent's attack. Even the Li is strong, it is useless.

倘能以十斤之勁，集於手而中於人，人必傷。數十
斤之勁，集於足而中於人，人必斃。則亦何患乎力
之不多也。他拳之勢，掌則為掌，肘則為肘，顯然
易知。然學者積久成習，尚多有粗疏木強，不能集
中其勁以達於敵人者，病在知有力之為力，不知無
力之為力也。握拳透爪，齧齒穿齦，自視殊武健，
而不知力因此已陷於肩背，徒為他人攻擊之藉，力
雖大何補。

The principle of Taijiquan is to transform the Li into Jin, especially can concentrate as wish. When it is used, it is working and when it is not used, it can be hidden. There is no sickness of coarseness, stiffness, and hardness and no trace of bending, extending, breaking, and continuing. Therefore, the classic says: 'Those without the Qi are pure hard.' That means do not use the Li, not without using the Jin."

太極拳之原則，在化力為勁，尤在能任意集中。用
之則行，舍之則藏，無粗疏木強之弊，無屈伸斷續
之跡。故經曰：「無氣者純剛。」是不用力也，非
不用勁也。」

The guest said: "Truly as you said. Then, I have studied (and practiced) day and night for three years, have never been not slow, and never use the force, how come I cannot defeat (my opponent) even once?"

客曰：「誠如吾子之說，則吾三年來寢饋其中，未
嘗不慢，未嘗用力，何為而不得一當也？」

I said: "The ancient people derived the theory so as to create the postures. (Therefore), we should be able to

*understand the theory from the postures. Without know-
ing the theory and simply training the postures, even
other fists cannot be achieved, not even mention the
deep and profound Taijiquan. Even practiced for thirty
years, it will still not be useful."*

余曰：〝古人緣理以造勢，吾人應即勢以明理。不
知理而徒練勢，他拳且不可，況精深博大之太極拳
乎。雖寢處其中三十年，亦何益也。〞

*The guest said: "Then, how can it be done so it can be
useful?"*

客曰：〝然則如何而後可？〞

*I said: "(If) training the body (i.e., postures), then rely
on mastering the theory of the ancient classics and place
all of the effort to experience it. If training the applications, then study and play (i.e., practice) the classic:*
Song of Striking and Training Comprehension of the
Thirteen Postures, *then, it can be done.*

余曰：〝練體、惟熟讀經論，力求體驗。練用、則
玩索打手歌，及十三勢行功心解，斯亦可矣。〞

*The guest said: "(I) did not wait for what you said
and have engaged on studying them already in the
past. Talking about theory, from mastering and gradually comprehending the understanding Jin, from under-*

standing Jin gradually reaching the enlightenment. I studied nearly thirty times daily. The techniques written (in the classics) cannot said not familiar already. Three years have passed, my effort in it cannot be said not long. However, I cannot see the effectiveness of the sudden comprehension. Therefore, I doubt about it."

客曰：「是不待吾子之命。曩嘗從事於斯矣。論言、由著熟漸悟懂勁，由懂勁階及神明。吾日習幾三十遍，著法不為不熟矣。為時三年，用力不為不久矣。而豁然貫通之效不見，是以疑之。」

I said: "What you said about mastering, are those (skills) which can be manifested externally as advance, retreat, or circling? If (you) can know the Yi (i.e., intention or wisdom mind) and discriminate insubstantial and substantial clearly, then the more you practice the postures, the more refined the Yi (is developed). What is said to transport the Qi as in a nine-curved pearl, no place cannot be reached. Then entire body, four limbs, and hundred skeletons, no place cannot store the Jin and no place cannot emit the Jin. That means (I am) able to yield wherever and able to stick wherever. In this case, how can you be defeated by those who learned other fists (i.e., styles) only a few months?"

余曰：「子之所謂著熟者，殆其形於外之進退周旋歟。若能心知其意，虛實分明，則勢愈練而意愈縝密。所謂行氣如九曲珠，無微不至。則一身之四肢百骸，無在不可以蓄勁，無在不可以發勁。即是隨處能走，隨處能粘。復安有敗退於學他拳才數月者之理。」

At this moment, the guest suddenly comprehended and said: "There is no definite timing for insubstantial and substantial, no definite positions. Use the Yi to vary (the situations). In theory, it is clear now. (However), when (I) apply the theory in the real situation, (I) always suffer because there is no base in advancing and retreating. Even sometimes (I) resist without feeling it. The sickness (i.e., problem) of double weighting is as if born naturally. It is hard to avoid (this problem). It is not because I do not know the problems are the insubstantial and substantial are not discriminated and the feeling is not acute (i.e., sensitive). However, sometimes even (I) know how it should be, but cannot apply it (in the techniques). Is there any other reason for this?"

客至是恍然若有所悟，曰：〝虛實無定時，無定位，以意為變化，於理則然矣。施之於事，每苦進退失據，甚且頂抗蠻觸於不自覺。雙重之病，有若天性使然，避之甚難。吾非不知病在虛實未分明也。觸覺未敏銳也。然有時明知其然，而法無可施者，其故亦別有在乎？〞

I said: "Among the thirteen postures, the central equilibrium is the major (i.e., most important). Other twelve postures such as Peng, Lu, Ji, An are assistant. (Only if) there is a central equilibrium, then can have everything. All of the postures cannot be separated from central equilibrium. Only then, (you) can talk about how to deal with (the situation). Chen, Ping-San said that opening, closing, insubstantial, and substantial are the fist classic (i.e., fist theory). We should understand that if there is no central equilibrium, how can it have opening and closing. It is just like the door and window, its opening and closing are on the hinge. If the hinge is loose, how can you open and close. If not able to open and close, how can the insubstantial and substantial be originated? Therefore, it is understood that the insubstantial and substantial without central equilibrium, it is not real insubstantial and substantial. (If) there is no feeling of central equilibrium, it is like the vision of blindness, the walking of a cripple, touch as without touching, and feel as without feeling. The classic said: 'Center, upright, peace, and comfortable.' The peace and comfortable is what is the equilibrium."

余曰：〝十三勢以中定為主，掤攦擠按十二勢為輔。有中定，然後有一切。一切勢皆不離乎中定，然後足以言應付。陳品三謂開闔虛實，即為拳經。吾人應知無中定，安有開闔。譬之戶牖，開闔在樞。樞若動搖，云何開闔。不開不闔，虛實焉求。是可知無中定之虛實，非虛實也·無中定之觸覺，猶瞽之視，跛之履，觸如不觸，覺如不覺也。經曰：中正安舒´，安舒云者，定之謂也。〞

The guest said: "Is there a Dao (i.e., method) for reaching the central equilibrium?"

客曰：〝求中定有道乎？〞

I said: "You only know that the insubstantial and substantial do not have definite timing and definite position, and use the Yi as a variable (factor for any change). But (you) do not know in every insubstantial and substantial, there must first be central equilibrium, then there is a variation. (That means), everywhere has the insubstantial and substantial, then everywhere has the central equilibrium. It is because the methods (i.e., techniques) do not have a definite position, and all of the methods are derived from central equilibrium. Even the holy man is reborn, (he) will not change what I have said. The methods are applied to the entire body, then the central equilibrium is also applied in the entire body. However, it is not easy to talk about this with beginners. Nevertheless, when searching for the opening and the closing of the left and the right, the hinge (i.e., key) is on the spine. The hinge of the up and down opening and closing is on the waist.

余曰：「子但知虛實無定時，無定位，以意為變化
。而不知每一虛實，皆先有中定，而後有變化。處
處有虛實，即處處有中定。蓋法無定位，而一切法
皆從中定中出。則聖人復起，不易吾言也。法遍周
身，中定亦遍周身。然初學者，不足以語此。無己
，則求左右開闔之樞，在脊，上下開闔之樞，在腰
。

The ancestor said the Li (i.e., power) was originated from the spine, what was said about the tailbone is upright, what was said the Qi (circulates) following the back and condense the Qi into the spine bone, what was said the head is suspended, all of these clearly imply the hinge (i.e., crucial keys) are on the spine. What was said the waist is like a car's axle, what was said the waist is like a banner, what was said the life and the Yi's origins are on the waist, what is said pay attention to the waist every moment, what was said mastered by the waist, all clearly point out that the hinge (i.e., the key) is on the waist. The learner therefore must first aim for the central equilibrium of the waist and spine, only then can all of the techniques have the central equilibrium. If not doing so, even practice since the childhood until the hair is white (i.e., old) will still be in vain. The song of thirteen postures said: 'If not

*aiming for this (i.e., central equilibrium), then (you)
will sigh of wasting Gongfu (i.e., energy-time).' Alas!
All of these sayings from the wise ancestors, as if their
voices can be heard."*

先哲所謂力由脊發，所謂尾閭正中，所謂氣貼背斂
入脊骨，所謂頂頭懸，皆明示其樞在脊也。所謂腰
如車軸，所謂腰為纛，所謂命意源頭在腰際，所謂
刻刻留心在腰間，所謂主宰於腰，皆明示其樞在腰
也。學者先求得腰脊之中定，然後一切法，乃有中
定。非然者，雖童而習之，以至於皓首，猶無益也
。十三勢歌云：「若不向此推求去，枉費工夫貽嘆
息。」嗚呼，昔賢悲憫之言，如聞其聲矣。"

*The guest listened and bowed (to me) again and said:
"Seldom hear your talking (i.e., teaching). Though I
study the classic and theses everyday, still cannot grasp
its gap (i.e., essence). However, (I) have more questions
to ask you. The classic said the Qi should be full and
drumming like a drum, the Qi is sunken to the (Lower)
Dan Tian. The Song of the Thirteen Postures said:
'circulate the Qi around the entire body without slight
stagnation.' Training Comprehension of the Thirteen
Postures said: 'Use the Xin (i.e., emotional mind) to
transport the Qi and use the Qi to function the body.'
Many of these talk about Qi. However, what is the
method to make the Qi full as a drum, to make the
Qi sunken to the Dan Tian, to circulate the Qi to the
entire body and limbs. Xin, how does it lead the Qi?
How can the Qi activate the (physical body). Though
(I) know clearly that these (theories) are the crucial
keys, however, (I) am suffered that (I) don't know where
to begin. Furthermore, Dan Tian locates below the
navel. According to today's scientists, said: the breathing uses the lungs not abdomen. The breathing cannot
reach the (place) below diaphragm. What is called the*

abdominal breathing is actually only the exercises of the diaphragm. What method can lead the Qi sunken to the Dan Tian?"

客聞而再拜曰：〝微吾子言，吾雖日讀經論，而不
得間也。抑更有請者。經言氣宜鼓盪，論言，氣沉
丹田。十三勢歌言，氣遍身軀不少滯。十三勢行功
心解言，以心行氣，以氣運身。其言氣者多矣。究
竟氣以何法使鼓盪，使沉丹田，使遍身軀。心、如
何行氣。氣如何運身。明知氣為此中肝要，然苦無
下手處。且丹田在臍以下。今之理學家，謂呼吸以
肺不以腹，橫膈膜以下，非呼吸所能達。所謂腹部
呼吸者，橫膈膜之運動而已。其將以何法使氣沉丹
田？〞

I said: "Good question you have asked. If a person gives up his breathing, then without the air (i.e., oxygen). What is called the Qi is sunken to the Dan Tian means the Yi (i.e., wisdom mind) is kept at the Dan Tian. It is what is meant inside the abdomen is relaxed and calm, and the Qi is abundantly raising. Every moment pay attention to the waist. Those who practice Taijiquan should aim that in every opening and closing of the posture, the Xin is there and the Yi is investigating the opponent's Yi (i.e., intention), then use the breathing to decorate (i.e., coordinate and harmonize) in the opening and closing. Exhalation is for opening and inhalation is for closing. In every posture, there is the foot's opening and closing, the body's opening and closing, the up-down and left-right's opening and closing, the internal and external's opening and closing. Every opening and closing is one exhalation and inhalation. Where is the opening and closing is where is the Yi. After practicing for a long lime, naturally the Qi will circulate around the entire body. Where to start to train this Gong (i.e., Gongfu) is on the breathing. To achieve the unbelievable marvellous Gong is also on the breathing. In the classic, Training Comprehension of the Thirteen Postures, *it is said: 'can breathe, then can be agile and alive.' This is what is meant."*

余曰：〝善哉問乎。夫人捨呼吸外無氣。所謂氣沉丹田，即意存丹田也，亦即所謂腹內鬆靜氣騰然，刻刻留心在腰際也。習太極拳者，求每勢之開闔。勢勢存心，揆其用意，然後以呼吸麗於開闔之中。呼為開，吸為闔。各勢中有手開闔，足開闔，身開闔，縱橫開闔，內外開闔，一開闔即一呼吸。開闔所在，即意所在。習之既久，自然氣遍周身。下手之功在呼吸，成就玄妙不思議之功，亦在呼吸。行功心解中，謂能呼吸，而後能靈活，此也。〞

The guest said: "Many people have read the Taijiquan classics. However, actually it is very hard to find those who are really able to comprehend deeply in the heart and gather the spirit without any obstacles (i.e., difficulty in understanding). You should write a book and discuss what we have just discussed, so it can show the upcoming (Taijiquan practitioners) a correct path. Can this also be used to untie the doubts for those who study this Dao (i.e., Taijiquan)?"

客曰：〝讀太極拳經論者多矣。果能心領神會，事理無礙者，實未易多覯。吾子盍書適所論列者，以昭式來茲，或亦足為研習此道者解惑之一助歟？〞

I said: "Yes. The Taijiquan instructor Mr. Wu, Yu-Ting (nickname of Wu, Gong-Zao) in Hunan Guoshu Training Institute, who inherited his father, Mr. Jian-Quan's techniques and is renowned at this time. He has also compiled and written this book: The Lecture of Taijiquan. *We can find other writings, that only contain pictures without any explanation of essential meaning (of Taijiquan). In addition, they include the subject of the five elements, eight trigrams, and deep and hard to understand theory of Yi (i.e., book of change), which are not even related to the art (i.e., Taijiquan). Naturally, there is as big a difference as the heaven and the earth. (Mr. Wu) asked me to write a foreword for him. I have felt sad that this Dao (i.e., Taijiquan) has never been correctly understood. It just happened that I should have a discussion with a guest. These subjects are not discussed in detail in Mr. Wu's writings. Therefore, I write this foreword for his book.*

余曰：〝唯。湖南國術訓練所太極拳教官吳雨亭君，能傳其父鍵泉先生之術，有聲於時，並為諸生編太極拳術講義。以視當世僅注圖解，毫無當於精義。或摭拾五行八卦與藝術無關之艱深易理諸著作，自有天壤之別。責序於余。余久悲此道之難有正知見也。與客適所論列，復為吳著所不詳。是書以歸之。是為序。〞

June, 1937, Ping-Jiang, Xiang, Kai-Ran
民國二十六年六月平江向愷然序

Appendix B
Translation and Glossary of Chinese Terms

An 安

Means "peace."

An 按

Means "pressing or stamping." One of the eight basic moving or Jin patterns of Taijiquan. These eight moving patterns are called "Ba Men" (八門) which means "eight doors." When An is done, first relax the wrist and when the hand has reached the opponent's body, immediately settle down the wrist. This action is called "Zuo Wan" (坐腕) in Taijiquan practice.

An Jin 按勁

The martial power generated from the An moving pattern of Taijiquan.

Bagua (Ba Kua) 八卦

Literally, "Eight Divinations." Also called the Eight Trigrams. In Chinese philosophy, the eight basic variations; shown in the Yi Jing (易經)(Book of Change) as groups of single and broken lines.

Ba Men Wu Bu 八門五步

Means "eight doors and five steppings." The art of Taijiquan is constructed from eight basic moving or Jin patterns and the five basic steppings. The eight basic moving or Jin patterns that can be used to handle the eight directions of action are called the "eight doors" (Ba Men, 八門) and the five stepping actions are called the "five steppings" (Wu Bu, 五步).

Bai He 白鶴

"White Crane." A style of Chinese martial arts.

Bu Diu Bu Ding 不丢不頂

"Do not lose contact and do no resist." A Taijiquan key phrase about adhering and following.

Cai 採

"Plucking."

Cai Jin 採勁

The martial power of plucking.

Chang Chuan (Changquan) 長拳

Means "long range fist or "long sequence." Chang Chuan includes all northern Chinese long range martial styles. Taijiquan is also called Chang Chuan simply because its sequence is long.

Changquan (Chang Chuan) 長拳

Means "long range fist" or "long sequence." Chang Chuan includes all northern Chinese long range martial styles. Taijiquan is also called Chang Chuan simply because its sequence is long.

Cheng, Gin-Gsao (1911-1976 A.D.) 曾金灶

Dr. Yang, Jwing-Ming's White Crane master.

Chi (Qi) 氣

The energy pervading the universe, including the energy circulating in the human body.

Chi Kung (Qigong) 氣功

The Gongfu of Qi, which means the study of Qi.

Chin Na (Qin Na) 擒拿

Literally means "seize control." A component of Chinese martial arts which emphasizes grabbing techniques, to control your opponent's joints, in conjunction with attacking certain acupuncture cavities.

Dan Tian 丹田

Literally: "Field of Elixir." Locations in the body which are able to store and generate Qi (elixir) in the body. The Upper, Middle, and Lower Dan Tians are located respectively between the eyebrows, at the solar plexus, and a few inches below the navel.

Dian Xue 點穴

Dian means "to point and exert pressure" and Xue means "the cavities." Dian Xue refers to those Qin Na techniques which specialize in attacking acupuncture cavities to immobilize or kill an opponent.

Dian Xue massages 點穴按摩

Cavity press massage.

Dong Jin 懂勁

"Understanding Jin." One of the Jins which uses the feeling of the skin to sense the opponent's energy.

Dui 兌

One of the Eight Trigrams.

Gen 艮

One of the Eight Trigrams. It represents mountains.

Gong (Kung) 功

Energy or hard work.

Gongfu (Kung Fu) 功夫

Means "energy-time." Anything which will take time and energy to learn or to accomplish is called Gongfu.

Han, Ching-Tang 韓慶堂

A well known Chinese martial artist, especially in Taiwan in the last forty years. Master Han is also Dr. Yang Jwing-Ming's Long Fist grandmaster.

Hua Jin 化勁

The Jin (martial power) used to neutralize the opponent's attacking.

Huan Jing Bu Nao 還精補腦

Literally, to return the Essence to nourish the brain. A Daoist Qigong training process wherein Qi which has been converted from Essence is lead to the brain to nourish it.

Huang Ting 黃庭

"Yellow yard." 1. A yard or hall in which Daoists, who often wore yellow robes, meditate together. 2. In Daoist Qigong, the place in the center of the body where Fire Qi and Water Qi are mixed to generate a spiritual embryo.

Hubei Province 湖北省

One of the provinces in southern China.

Huo 火

Fire. One of the Five Elements.

Ji 擠

Means "to squeeze" or "to press."

Ji Jin 擠勁

The martial power of pressing or squeezing.

Jin 金

"Metal." One of the Five Elements.

Jin (Jing) 勁

Chinese martial power. A combination of "Li" (力)(muscular power) and "Qi" (氣).

Jin Bu 進步

"Step forward."

Jin, Shao-Feng 金紹峰

Master Yang Jwing-Ming's White Crane grandmaster.

Kan 坎

One of the Eight Trigrams, meaning "water." Referred to in "Kan and Li (fire)."

Kao 靠

Means "to lean or to press against." In Taijiquan, it means to bump someone off balance.

Kao Jin 靠勁

The martial power of bumping.

Kao, Tao 高濤

Dr. Yang, Jwing-Ming's first Taijiquan master.

Kun 坤

One of the Eight Trigrams.

Kung (Gong) 功

Means "energy" or "hard work."

Kung Fu (Gongfu) 功夫

Means "energy-time." Anything which will take time and energy to learn or to accomplish is called Kung Fu.

Li 離

One of the Eight Trigrams, meaning "fire." Referred to in "Kan (water) and Li."

Li, Mao-Ching 李茂清

Dr. Yang, Jwing-Ming's Long Fist master.

Lian 連

"To connect."

Lian Jin 連勁

The martial power of connecting.

Liang Yi 兩儀

"Two Poles." It means Yin and Yang.

Lie 挒

Means "to rend" or "to split."

Lie Jin 挒勁

The martial power of "split" or "rend."

Lu 擺

Means "to rollback."

Lu Jin 擺勁

The martial power of rolling backward (rollback).

Ma, Yue-Liang 馬岳梁

A well-known Wu Style Taijiquan master. Wu, Jian-Quan's son-in-law.

Mi 米

"Rice."

Mu 木

"Wood." One of the Five Elements.

Nei Jia 內家

Literally, "internal family." It implies "internal martial styles."

Nei Jin 內勁

"Internal Jin." Means the concentrated mind leading the Qi for physical manifestation.

Nian 黏

To stick or to adhere.

Nian Jin 黏勁

The martial power of adhering.

Pan Jia 盤架

Means "entwine the frame" in Chinese. It is common terminology in Chinese martial arts. At the beginning of your practice, you learn how to squat down to firm your root (i.e., fundamental stances) and to practice the basic physical movements to build up a foundation. All of these trainings are called "Pan Jia."

Peng 掤

Means "to ward off."

Peng Jin 掤勁

The martial power of warding off.

Qian 乾

One of the Eight Trigrams.

Qigong (Chi Kung) 氣功

The Gongfu of Qi, which means the study of Qi.

Qin Na (Chin Na) 擒拿

Literally means "seize control." A component of Chinese martial arts which emphasizes grabbing techniques to control your opponent's joints, in conjunction with attacking certain acupuncture cavities.

Quan Shu 拳術

Literally, "fist techniques" and means martial arts.

San Shi Qi Shi 三十七勢

"Thirty-seven postures." Yang Style Taijiquan is also called Thirty-seven postures since it is constructed by thirty-seven fundamental movements.

Shaolin 少林

A Buddhist temple in Henan Province, famous for its martial arts.

Shi San Shi 十三勢

"Thirteen Patterns." Taijiquan is also called Shi San Shi since the art of Taijiquan is constructed from these thirteen moving or acting patterns.

Shuang Zhong 雙重

Means "double weighting or double layering." It means when the opponent has placed a weight or pressure on you, you respond by meeting that pressure with equal or greater pressure of your own. The consequence is stagnation. When this happens, mutual resistance will be generated.

Shui 水

"Water." One of the Five Elements.

Si Xiang 四象

Means "Four Phases" which are derived from Two Poles.

Sui 隨

Means "to follow."

Sui Jin 隨勁

"Following Jin." The martial power which is used to follow the opponent's action.

Sun Wu 孫武

Also named as Sun Zi (孫子). A famous strategist who lived around 557 B.C. He wrote a book: *Sun Zi's Fighting Strategies* (Sun Zi Bing Fa, 孫子兵法). This book is commonly translated as *"The Art of War."*

Sun Zi 孫子

"Mister Sun." Sun Wu (孫武). A famous strategist who lived around 557 B.C. He wrote a book: *Sun Zi's Fighting Strategies* (*Sun Zi Bing Fa,* 孫子兵法). This book is commonly translated as *"The Art of War."*

Sun Zi Bing Fa 孫子兵法

"Sun Zi's Fighting Strategies". Name of a book which is commonly translated as *"The Art of War."*

Tai Chi Chuan (Taijiquan) 太極拳

A Chinese internal martial style which is based on the theory of Taiji (grand ultimate).

Taiji 太極

Means "grand ultimate." It is this force which generates two poles, Yin and Yang.

Taijiquan (Tai Chi Chuan) 太極拳

A Chinese internal martial style which is based on the theory of Taiji (grand ultimate).

Taipel 台北

The capital city of Taiwan located in the north of Taiwan.

Taipei Xian 台北縣

A county in northern Taiwan.

Taiwan 台灣

An island to the southeast of mainland China. Also known as "Formosa."

Taiwan University 台灣大學

A well-known university located in Taipei, Taiwan.

Taizuquan 太祖拳

A style of Chinese external martial arts.

Tamkang 淡江

Name of a University in Taiwan.

Tamkang College Guoshu Club 淡江國術社

A Chinese martial arts club founded by Dr. Yang when he was studying in Tamkang College.

Tiao 調

A gradual regulating process resulting in that which is regulated achieving harmony with others.

Tiao Qi 調氣

To regulate the Qi.

Tiao Shen 調神

To regulate the spirit.

Tiao Shen 調身

To regulate the body.

Tiao Xi 調息

To regulate the breathing.

Tiao Xin 調心

To regulate the emotional mind.

Ting 聽

"Listening."

Ting Jin 聽勁

"Listening Jin." A special training which uses the skin to feel the opponent's energy and from this feeling to further understand his intention.

Tu 土

"Earth." One of the Five Elements.

Tui Bu 退步

"Step backward." One of the five basic steppings in Taijiquan.

Tui Na 推拿

Means "to push and grab." A category of Chinese massages for healing and injury treatment.

Wai Jin 外勁

"External Jin." The external body movements of the Jin's manifestation.

Wang, Zong-Yue 王宗岳

A well-known Taijiquan master during the late Qing Dynasty. Wang, Zong-Yue wrote many comprehensive Taijiquan documents and is popularly studied by Taijiquan practitioners today.

Wilson Chen 陳威伸

Dr. Yang, Jwing-Ming's martial art friend.

Wu Bu 五步

"Five steppings." They include: forward, backward, left, right, and center.

Wu Style Taijiquan 吳氏太極拳

A style of Taijiquan created by Wu, Quan-You (吳全佑)(1834-1902).

Wu, Gong-Yi 吳公儀

Wu, Jian-Quan's son.

Wu, Gong-Zao 吳公藻

Wu, Jian-Quan's son who wrote a book: *The Lecture of Taijiquan,* (太極拳講義),1935, Shanghai, China.

Wu, Jian-Quan (1870-1942) 吳鑑泉

The second generation of Wu Style Taijiquan.

Wu, Jun-Hua 吳俊華

Wu, Jian-Quan's daughter.

Wu, Quan-You (1834-1902) 吳全佑

The creator of Wu Style Taijiquan who learned Taijiquan from Yang, Ban-Hou (楊班候)(1837-1892).

Wu, Ying-Hua 吳英華

Wu, Jian-Quan's daughter.

Wuxing 五行

Five Elements, including Metal, Wood, Water, Fire, and Earth.

Wudang Mountain 武當山

Located in Hubei Province (湖北省) in China.

Wuji 無極

Means "no extremity."

Wushu 武術

Literally, "martial techniques."

Xiang, Kai-Ran (1889-1957 A.D.) 向愷然

A famous Taijiquan master, also named Xiang, Kui (向逵), nick-named Bu Xiao Sheng (不肖生); Ancestors were living at Ping Jiang, Hunan Province (湖南‧平江). However, he was born at Xiang Tan (湘潭). He liked Wushu since he was young and was also interested in scholarship. First, he learned Wu family style (巫家拳) Wushu. In 1905 he went to Japan to study politics and law. While he was in Japan, he practiced Wushu with a Chinese student Wang, Zhi-Qun (王志群). In 1911, he returned to China and was employed as a military judge in Chang Sa (長沙). In 1913, he again went to Japan to study in the Japanese Central University in Tokyo (日本東京中央大學). After he returned from Japan in 1917, he founded "The Chinese Fist Techniques Research Institute" (中華拳術研究會). He has written many books and novels such as: Fist Techniques (拳術), The Passage of Fist Techniques (拳術傳薪錄), The Seeing and Hearing of Fist Techniques (拳術見聞), etc.

Xin 心

Means "heart." Xin means the mind generated from emotional disturbance.

Xinzhu Xian 新竹縣

Birthplace of Dr. Yang, Jwing-Ming in Taiwan.

Xun 巽

One of the Eight Trigrams which represents "wind."

Yang 陽

Too sufficient. One of the two poles. The other is Yin.

Yang, Ban-Hou (1837-1892 A.D.) 楊班侯

Yang, Lu-Shan's second son. Also called Yang, Yu (楊鈺).

Yang, Jwing-Ming 楊俊敏

Author of this book.

Yang, Lu-Shan (1799-1872) 楊露禪

The creator of Yang Style Taijiquan.

Yang, Yu (1837-1892 A.D.) 楊鈺

Yang, Lu-Shan's second son. Also called Ban-Hou (班侯). A second generation practitioner of Yang style Taijiquan.

Yang Style Taijiquan 楊氏太極拳

A style of Taijiquan created by Yang, Lu-Shan (1799-1872).

Yi 意

"Wisdom mind." The mind generated from wise judgment.

Yi Jing 易經

"*Book of Changes.*" A book of divination written during the Zhou Dynasty (1122-255 B.C., 周).

Yin 陰

Deficient. One of the two poles. The other is Yang.

You Pan 右盼

"Look to the right."

Zhan 占

"To occupy."

Zhan 沾

"Attaching."

Zhan 粘

"Attaching" or "sticking."

Zhan Jin 粘勁

The martial power that is used to attack the opponent's body.

Zhang, San-Feng 張三豐

Zhang, San-Feng is credited as the creator of Taijiquan during the Song Dynasty in China (960-1127 A.D.)(宋朝).

Zhang, Xiang-San 張祥三

A well-known martial artist in Taiwan during the 1960's.

Zhen 震

One of the Eight Trigrams which represents "thunder."

Zhong Ding 中定

To firm the center.

Zhou 肘

"Elbow."

Zhou Jin 肘勁

The martial power generated from the elbow.

Zuo Gu 左顧

"Beware of the left."

Zuo Wan 坐腕

"Settle down the wrist."

Index

BOOKS FROM YMAA

6 HEALING MOVEMENTS
101 REFLECTIONS ON TAI CHI CHUAN
A WOMAN'S QIGONG GUIDE
ADVANCING IN TAE KWON DO
ANCIENT CHINESE WEAPONS
ANALYSIS OF SHAOLIN CHIN NA 2ND ED.
ARTHRITIS RELIEF — CHINESE QIGONG FOR HEALING &
     PREVENTION, 3RD ED.
BACK PAIN RELIEF — CHINESE QIGONG FOR HEALING & PREVENTION
     2ND ED
BAGUAZHANG
CARDIO KICKBOXING ELITE
CHIN NA IN GROUND FIGHTING
CHINESE FAST WRESTLING — THE ART OF SAN SHOU KUAI JIAO
CHINESE FITNESS — A MIND / BODY APPROACH
CHINESE TUI NA MASSAGE
COMPLETE CARDIOKICKBOXING
COMPREHENSIVE APPLICATIONS OF SHAOLIN CHIN NA
DUKKHA — A SAM REEVES MARTIAL ARTS THRILLER
EIGHT SIMPLE QIGONG EXERCISES FOR HEALTH, 2ND ED.
ESSENCE OF SHAOLIN WHITE CRANE
ESSENCE OF TAIJI QIGONG, 2ND ED.
EXPLORING TAI CHI
FACING VIOLENCE
FIGHTING ARTS
INSIDE TAI CHI
KATA AND THE TRANSMISSION OF KNOWLEDGE
LITTLE BLACK BOOK OF VIOLENCE
LIUHEBAFA FIVE CHARACTER SECRETS
MARTIAL ARTS ATHLETE
MARTIAL ARTS INSTRUCTION
MARTIAL WAY AND ITS VIRTUES
MEDITATIONS ON VIOLENCE
MIND/BODY FITNESS — A MIND / BODY APPROACH
MUGAI RYU — THE CLASSICAL SAMURAI ART OF DRAWING THE
     SWORD
NATURAL HEALING WITH QIGONG — THERAPEUTIC QIGONG
NORTHERN SHAOLIN SWORD, 2ND ED.
OKINAWA'S COMPLETE KARATE SYSTEM — ISSHIN RYU
PRINCIPLES OF TRADITIONAL CHINESE MEDICINE
QIGONG FOR HEALTH & MARTIAL ARTS 2ND ED.
QIGONG FOR LIVING
QIGONG FOR TREATING COMMON AILMENTS

QIGONG MASSAGE —FUNDAMENTAL TECHNIQUES FOR HEALTH AND
     RELAXATION, 2ND ED.
QIGONG MEDITATION — EMBRYONIC BREATHING
QIGONG MEDITATION—SMALL CIRCULATION
QIGONG, THE SECRET OF YOUTH
QUIET TEACHER
ROOT OF CHINESE QIGONG, 2ND ED.
SHIN GI TAI—KARATE TRAINING FOR BODY, MIND, AND SPIRIT
SHIHAN TE — THE BUNKAI OF KATA
SUNRISE TAI CHI
SURVIVING ARMED ASSAULTS
TAEKWONDO — ANCIENT WISDOM FOR THE MODERN WARRIOR
TAEKWONDO — DEFENSE AGAINST WEAPONS
TAE KWON DO — THE KOREAN MARTIAL ART
TAEKWONDO — SPIRIT AND PRACTICE
TAI CHI BALL QIGONG—FOR HEALTH AND MARTIAL ARTS
TAI CHI BOOK
TAI CHI CHUAN — 24 & 48 POSTURES
TAI CHI CHUAN MARTIAL APPLICATIONS, 2ND ED.
TAI CHI CONNECTIONS
TAI CHI DYNAMICS
TAI CHI SECRETS OF THE ANCIENT MASTERS
TAI CHI SECRETS OF THE WU & LI STYLES
TAI CHI SECRETS OF THE YANG STYLE
TAI CHI THEORY & MARTIAL POWER, 2ND ED.
TAI CHI WALKING
TAIJI CHIN NA
TAIJI SWORD, CLASSICAL YANG STYLE
TAIJIQUAN, CLASSICAL YANG STYLE
TAIJIQUAN THEORY OF DR. YANG, JWING-MING
THE CROCODILE AND THE CRANE
THE CUTTING SEASON
THE WAY OF KATA—A COMPREHENSIVE GUIDE TO DECIPHERING
     MARTIAL APPS.
THE WAY OF KENDO AND KENJITSU
THE WAY OF SANCHIN KATA
THE WAY TO BLACK BELT
TRADITIONAL CHINESE HEALTH SECRETS
TRADITIONAL TAEKWONDO—CORE TECHNIQUES, HISTORY, AND
     PHILOSOPHY
WESTERN HERBS FOR MARTIAL ARTISTS
WILD GOOSE QIGONG
XINGYIQUAN, 2ND ED.

DVDS FROM YMAA

ANALYSIS OF SHAOLIN CHIN NA
ADVANCED PRACTICAL CHIN NA IN DEPTH
BAGUAZHANG 1,2, & 3 —EMEI BAGUAZHANG
CHEN STYLE TAIJIQUAN
CHIN NA IN DEPTH COURSES 1 — 4
CHIN NA IN DEPTH COURSES 5 — 8
CHIN NA IN DEPTH COURSES 9 — 12
EIGHT SIMPLE QIGONG EXERCISES FOR HEALTH
THE ESSENCE OF TAIJI QIGONG
FIVE ANIMAL SPORTS
KNIFE DEFENSE—TRADITIONAL TECHINIQUES AGAINST DAGGER
QIGONG FOR HEALING
QIGONG MASSAGE—FUNDAMENTAL TECHNIQUES FOR HEALTH AND
     RELAXATION
SHAOLIN KUNG FU FUNDAMENTAL TRAINING 1&2
SHAOLIN LONG FIST KUNG FU — BASIC SEQUENCES
SHAOLIN SABER — BASIC SEQUENCES
SHAOLIN STAFF — BASIC SEQUENCES
SHAOLIN WHITE CRANE GONG FU BASIC TRAINING 1&2
SIMPLE QIGONG EXERCISES FOR ARTHRITIS RELIEF
SIMPLE QIGONG EXERCISES FOR BACK PAIN RELIEF
SIMPLIFIED TAI CHI CHUAN
SUNRISE TAI CHI
SUNSET TAI CHI
SWORD—FUNDAMENTAL TRAINING

TAI CHI ENERGY PATTERNS
TAIJI BALL QIGONG COURSES 1&2—16 CIRCLING AND 16 ROTATING
     PATTERNS
TAIJI BALL QIGONG COURSES 3&4—16 PATTERNS OF WRAP-
     COILING & APPLICATIONS
TAIJI MARTIAL APPLICATIONS — 37 POSTURES
TAIJI PUSHING HANDS 1&2—YANG STYLE SINGLE AND DOUBLE
     PUSHING HANDS
TAIJI PUSHING HANDS 3&4—MOVING SINGLE AND DOUBLE PUSHING
     HANDS
TAIJI SABER — THE COMPLETE FORM, QIGONG & APPLICATIONS
TAIJI & SHAOLIN STAFF - FUNDAMENTAL TRAINING
TAIJI YIN YANG STICKING HANDS
TAIJIQUAN CLASSICAL YANG STYLE
TAIJI SWORD, CLASSICAL YANG STYLE
UNDERSTANDING QIGONG 1 — WHAT IS QI? • HUMAN QI CIRCULATORY
     SYSTEM
UNDERSTANDING QIGONG 2 — KEY POINTS • QIGONG BREATHING
UNDERSTANDING QIGONG 3 — EMBRYONIC BREATHING
UNDERSTANDING QIGONG 4 — FOUR SEASONS QIGONG
UNDERSTANDING QIGONG 5 — SMALL CIRCULATION
UNDERSTANDING QIGONG 6 — MARTIAL QIGONG BREATHING
WHITE CRANE HARD & SOFT QIGONG
YANG TAI CHI FOR BEGINNERS

more products available from...
YMAA Publication Center, Inc. 楊氏東方文化出版中心
1-800-669-8892 • info@ymaa.com • www.ymaa.com